Narcissistic Sibling

How to Recognize, Disarm, and
Shield Yourself from Narcissistic
Brothers and Sisters. Look Out
for Behavior Signs, and Learn to
Identify and Grasp the Covert
Narcissistic Personality Disorder

Mona Diggins

Table of Contents

Introduction

*"One thing a narcissist does not like is to look
in a mirror that is in any way genuinely
reflective of what's on the other side of it."*

—Jay Parini

Our televisions show us plenty of examples of how siblings are "supposed" to act. We see Tia and Tamera and their unique on-screen chemistry. We see the Hemsworth brothers looking fashionable and airbrushed on the red carpet. Even in fiction, we are shown sibling dynamics, such as the leading cast in *The Lion, the Witch, and the Wardrobe*, as they tackle their next adventure. The Weasleys in J. K. Rowling's *Harry Potter* are quirky and playful, Anna and Elsa of Disney's *Frozen* have each other's backs, and the Winchesters in CW's *Supernatural* share a deep brotherhood that saves the world time and time again.

Our media convincingly portrays siblinghood as an unconditional friendship that endures our lives' complexities and can inspire the people around us to love one another. It is a common trope. It leads many people who were born as the only child of their family to wish that they had a brother or sister to confide in, protect, and have quirky sleepovers with.

But sibling relationship is not always like that, is it?

Sometimes, being siblings means barely tolerating each other. Our siblings can disappoint us, make us jealous, hold us back, and make our living conditions a living hell. Even if we want to be like Anna and Elsa, reality never seems to fulfill the fantasy. No one expects a relationship to go smoothly 100 percent of the time or be identical to what we see in the movies. However, at what point does healthy sibling rivalry tip into the realm of narcissism?

Does your sibling constantly lie, especially when they see an opportunity to ruin your reputation and make you look like the bad guy? Do they blame you for everything that goes wrong, even if it is a situation that you have no direct control over? Is your sibling a personality chameleon capable of shaping their behaviors according to whoever is around them? Are they unrecognizable around their friends and value their image to an unhealthy degree? Have you tried talking to your sibling about these problems but were met with hostility, defensiveness, and even revenge? Have you developed trust issues, low self-esteem, and other trauma responses as a direct consequence of your sibling's actions?

Siblings can sometimes drive all of us up a wall, but those sorts of behaviors indicate a deeper issue. You should not be suffering from long-term symptoms just because you lived with a sibling for the first 20 or so years of your life. You should not have to worry about what your sibling has said about you to the people you care about. You should not be blamed for things you have not done. If this is the type of relationship you share with your sibling, they are likely a narcissist.

I know first-hand how difficult it is to live with a narcissist. I suffered abuse from a narcissist I co-parent with, so I understand the frustration and powerlessness that comes with handling that sort of personality. I know how it can drain you, ruin your self-image, and affect your future relationships. After dealing with this personality for many years, I knew I had to do something. I was determined to understand narcissism and other personality disorders to protect myself and help others in similar circumstances. I studied for five years to understand the psyche of a narcissist. The knowledge I have gained has been extremely helpful in improving the overall quality of my life. Now, I am writing this book in the hopes of helping those who are also forced to coexist with a narcissist.

We all have that one friend whose relationship advice is always the same: "Break up with them." You might even be that friend! That is fine; sometimes, breaking up is the right thing to do, and someone needs to say it. Unfortunately, however, cutting off unhealthy relationships is not always so simple. We do not choose our siblings, and although we might move away from them and create some distance, we will still have to interact with them in some way for the rest of our lives.

They will still be there during family events, holiday dinners, weddings, and plenty more. I know this well, so I am not here to tell you how to "break up" with your sibling. I am here to tell you how to live peacefully with them and protect yourself from their psychological attacks. Because I had to continue co-parenting with the narcissist in my life, I strived for coexistence rather than a complete door slam when I first began my studies. Therefore, I will help you obtain a similar sort of harmony with your sibling.

By the time you are done with this book, here are some of the things you will be able to do with ease:

- Understand the ins and outs of narcissism, its symptoms, and what causes it.
- Identify the types and subtypes of narcissism and determine which type best describes your sibling.
- Recognize the cycle of abuse, understand what stage you are in, and know the best course of action depending on where you are in the cycle.
- Realize the defining traits of a healthy relationship and see how they compare to your sibling dynamic.
- Know the motives behind narcissistic behaviors and label the characteristics of the disorder in real-life examples.
- Fight your feelings of guilt, blame, and burnout that you are experiencing after years of navigating manipulation.

- Use tools and techniques designed to help you discern manipulation from reality.
- Create healthy boundaries, limit contact, and develop other defense mechanisms while also keeping yourself safe from revenge plots and lies.
- Know some real-life stories from other people who have lived with narcissistic siblings.
- Avoid being made into the "bad guy" in every situation that inconveniences your sibling.
- Identify specific manipulation tactics, such as triangulation, so that you can avoid falling for your sibling's traps.
- Recover from the emotional trauma your sibling has put you through so that you can enjoy your other adult relationships with no baggage.
- Realize that you are not alone, that your struggles are valid, and that you are not powerless in this situation.
- Empower yourself and move on from this difficult stage of your life.
- Take all of that knowledge and apply it in a way that will keep you safe.

No more walking on eggshells, no more bending over backward to make your sibling happy. You may not be able to "fix" your sibling and make them a better person, but that is not your job in the first place. Your job is to keep yourself safe and ensure that you can have a happy future regardless of the person you shared a house with for the first few decades of your life. You will gain a greater sense of control and a sense of freedom that you haven't had since your sibling has begun engaging in narcissistic behaviors. Moreover, you will be able to do this without resorting to petty methods. You will remain polite but assertive.

As we enter the meat of the topic, allow me to explain some of the language that I will be using. You may have already noticed that I refer to your sibling in gender-neutral terms and use neutral pronouns when talking about them in the third person. I am choosing to do this because all genders can be narcissists, just as all genders can be victims of a narcissist. This issue also affects siblings of the same gender and siblings of different genders, so I will make no assumptions about your relationship in that regard. I will be using some anecdotal evidence throughout the book where I may mention the genders of the parties involved, but please assume that the behavior looks the same in all genders unless I specifically state otherwise. I will also avoid making assumptions about the rest of your family dynamic, so this book will be helpful for you regardless of your family. If anything I say is specific to a certain familial unit, I will state so.

Also, for the purpose of this book, I will only be discussing NPD (narcissistic personality disorder) and will only briefly touch on how the disorder may relate to other mental illnesses such as depression, anxiety, and so on. This book is meant as a general guide for understanding NPD and is not a tool for medical diagnosis of NPD or any other personality disorder. If you find that you need a medical diagnosis or want to pursue professional help for any reason, please seek out a therapist in your area. I will give specific tips on how to pursue therapy and what to expect once you start so that information will be available to you once we get there.

The key to fighting narcissistic behavior is to understand it, so we will begin with an in-depth description of the personality type. You will understand exactly why your narcissistic sibling puts up a front when they are talking to your family, friends, and peers. You will know how this front relates to their constant lies and exaggerations. You will know why your sibling may have developed NPD, what that means for the rest of your family, and how a therapist would likely deal with your sibling as a patient.

I know that it may feel counterproductive to start by empathizing with your narcissistic sibling and seeing things from their perspective. However, in truth, the extra knowledge will help you move forward in smart, decisive ways. As they say, knowledge is power! After you have grasped your narcissistic sibling's mindset, we will then move into practical tips that will allow you to disarm psychological attacks and give you a more solid ground to stand on. We will also discuss what to do as you move into the future and approach new relationships.

If you are ready to learn, empower, and take action, then go ahead and turn the page.

Chapter 1:

The Hidden Nature of

Narcissism

You have been here before, you tell yourself, glaring subtly over the rim of your glass while sitting down at another one of those unsettling family dinners. The entire experience is draining. Somehow, it always has been, even if you never quite understand why. Regardless, you have entertained some suspicions.

The target of your dagger-like stares: your narcissistic sibling. Whether they feel the sharp stab of your eyes seems inconsequential. They either taunt you to throw it their way or simply do not care. It drives you insane. In fact, this is not the first time you have questioned your sanity. Uncomfortable as the entire situation is, no one but you seems to notice—although someone besides you seems to know. You are looking at them. You have grown restless with the thought that the very reason for your discomfort is the person you are looking at. Still, the very idea of assigning blame to your brother or sister simply feels conflicting. Why then can't you shake the thought?

Perhaps the mounting evidence over the years has started to weigh too heavily on your mind. For one thing, you know that your every action is a strict exercise of self-control for the sake of preserving the peace. Calling them out on their charades have nearly ruined more than one family holiday, making you seem like the instigator to the conflict. So instead, you bite back your tongue. The effort, though, is exhausting. The alternative is a friendly conversation.

Engaging in peaceful banter with your sibling, however, seems like another monumental task. These conversations sometimes revolve in vicious circles that progressively confuse, disorientate, and make you question the views that you put across—even on simple things. The more you try to strengthen your standing on a topic, the more you are made to question its very premise. Your words seem to be tossed around like a salad, along with the nonsensical argument of your sibling. They never land as intended and always taste different from how you prepared them.

Not to mention that you dread being the center of any conversation—whether it be the object of someone's praise or the glaring spotlight of being looked upon to deliver an insight. In either case, you know that there is one person at that table who will try to steal your thunder without hesitation. The attention of others is an expensive commodity in your family, and your narcissistic sibling is out to claim it. It is greatly coveted that the very yearning for it has subjected you to a game you never wanted to be a part of—a survival of the fittest in the competition for attention.

However, your lion's share of attention becomes the scraps of assigned blame. Whether logical or not, the attention you are due is only when you are the scapegoat for your sibling's faults. Whether it be the neglectful arrangements communicated for that family dinner or the fight that inevitably ensues when the tension finally snaps over accusations at the dinner table, you are to blame. In fact, it is something your sibling makes certain of.

You have been an observer to some of these faults that your sibling adorns, almost like a badge. Suffice to say, you almost feel complicit in keeping some of it secret. Sitting at that dinner table, you wonder how to tell your parents of the deceptive dance your sibling has played with them. So many lies have been told—innocent when young, more serious with age—to cover up their misdeeds. For most of it, you may have convinced yourself that you were protecting them by keeping it a secret. However, now, you feel your help was always intended to be a smokescreen to their mistakes. The more you thought about it, the more you realized how you even felt coerced to offer to cover up for them, all for the sake of escaping what you dare not have said before—emotional abuse.

But how do you admit this—any of it—out loud (or even mention it) without sounding crazy? You recall the few times you have tried to address many of these situations. Still, in some way, you were made to question having ever held these suspicions and concerns in the first place. In some way, your words and motivations were twisted into intents that you never had. Through some outward or implicit tug at the strings, your narcissistic sibling managed to draw you out enough to voice confessions that make you seem unstable. They know how to play the puppeteer, but then again, have you been their puppet?

You feel unsettled at that dinner table, with the hoax of family harmony being the main course. You have found yourself in the precarious situation of keeping the peace while you were never a threat to it in the first place.

Yes, you have undoubtedly been here before. Perhaps you could never bring yourself to discover that you were breaking bread with a narcissist.

Of that bread, you have been biting away at the stale moments of self-doubt, guilt, and exhaustion that you forced yourself to swallow for more years than you would care to admit. To preserve your sanity, you accepted the conditions created by the orchestrator you could never bring yourself to credit for these feelings— your sibling. Despite the hardships of enduring their company, you could not bring yourself to call it out or find ways to disarm them. Their mind games have drained you, leaving you to reconcile with the pain in unsteady reflections.

It takes the truth to disarm doubt, and this truth comes from a knowledge that your sibling may not have even welcomed into their own understanding. It is the truth of what it means to be a narcissist and why you have been haunted by the unseen scars that have seemed so familiar despite the multiple efforts to discount their familiarity.

Narcissism is hard enough to identify. Your gut feeling tells you that something is genuinely amiss in your sibling interactions, but you have grown tired of the years of doubt it has afforded you. Recognizing and acknowledging the feelings stemming from your interactions with them is your most trustworthy source to implement change.

Your first move in reclaiming your power is knowing that the attempts at manipulation from your narcissistic sibling may be out of your control but your reaction to them is certainly not. Your feelings are way pointers to your actions, and subsequently, your feelings of discomfort should be seen as a warning sign. It is enough of a red flag that you can allow yourself to start contemplating what it really is about them that throws you off balance.

What Is Narcissism?

Family time may feel as though they are nothing short of vampiric. Past interactions with your narcissistic sibling around have left you spent in terms of acting as though everything is normal. You know that their life has been a series of deflecting blame and downplaying your success. They always fail to take accountability and continually violate your boundaries (Narcissistic Abuse Support, n.d.). Above that, you have been made to feel delusional for even highlighting these issues. However, allowing the truth of these feelings to set in is crucial to start looking for signs that your sibling may be a narcissist.

Your notion of these strained encounters is not unfounded. Narcissistic tendencies can be damaging to relationships, especially the family (Psychology Today, 2019). The family unit's tight-knit bonds offer the perfect rooting place for your sibling's narcissistic traits to be felt by others.

What, then, are these traits?

Firstly, you may have noticed an inflated sense of self-importance. Secondly, the grandiose nature of this leads them to think that they ultimately deserve special treatment. Thirdly, they may feel it should afford them a high degree of admiration from others. In fact, they need it. The only way they can get this is through seeking attention. Lastly, such beliefs pose a notable block toward any empathy they have for others. They should be the center of attention, and they want their needs to be always prioritized (Psychology Today, 2019).

Such exhibited characteristics are also not part of isolated events. If it had, your discomfort would not have led to seeking understanding. Instead, these habits form part of a consistent behavioral repertoire that you have seen play out over the years. If you do tie them to any specific event, it is likely part of your frame of reference that you can take as validation for your concerns.

It may have manifested in the many conversations about your respective careers. Somehow, despite the marginal evidence to support it, their job and achievements are always exaggerated above yours in a way that merits more attention. Despite the career milestones you may have achieved, you may feel that your narcissistic sibling deliberately downplays them every time you mention them in conversation. Then they will outshine them with their own remarkable successes. Somehow, the praise flows exactly where they intended—right into the infinite capacity of their admiration tank.

However, contrary to popular belief, the almost vampiric need for attention and the drive to have their appeal recognized due to grandiose beliefs is not always pathological. Narcissism only manifests on a clinical level in about 1 percent of the population. The most notable difference lies in the level of impairment it affords their daily functioning. Friction within their close personal relationships is often the strongest indicator in this regard (Psychology Today, 2019).

On a surface level, the pathological narcissist entertains bouts of admiration and pervasive ideations of power. Your sibling's needs to be applauded were not purely for the sake of gaining more attention. It had its purpose in contributing to their perceptions of power, whether through beauty, status, or success. It allowed them to feel superior, and consequently, it permitted them to feel entitled to this praise throughout their lives.

However, in the shadowy corners of their mind, the picture looks infinitely different. The outward need for attention almost becomes compensatory for the deep insecurities and sense of vulnerability. To protect themselves, they go to great lengths to attain what they think they need to fill the void within.

The History of Narcissistic Personality Disorder

In ancient Greece, the phenomenon of narcissism was called "hubris." It was associated with the stories of Icarus, Narcissus, and many more figures who were intended to dissuade people from prideful behavior and from disobeying the gods. In 1898, Havelock Ellis, an English sexologist, used the word "Narcissus-like" to describe the act of excessive masturbation and auto-eroticism, which he believed was rooted in a love for oneself. Since then, the Greek reference took off. The very next year, Paul Näche adjusted the wording and coined "narcissism" to refer to a similar phenomenon: sexual perversion.

However, it did not take long before narcissism became associated with something deeper and more involved than sexuality. In 1911, Otto Rank, Sigmund Freud's colleague, published the first psychoanalytical paper. It specifically focused on narcissism and its traits, which he identified as vanity and self-admiration.

Then, in 1914, Freud took this idea and published a paper of his own entitled *Narcissism: An Introduction.* His concept of narcissism differs a lot from our modern definition. He wanted to emphasize that some degree of narcissism is normal and necessary for our survival, drawing similarities to what we might call "self-preservation instincts." According to him, all healthy people have *primary narcissism* if they desire to stay alive. *Secondary narcissism* is when an individual has an excess of pridefulness that they had not matured out of from when they were young. In Freud's eyes, all children were narcissists, but they should have grown out of that phase as they grew older. People with secondary narcissism did not.

Freud's theory was fairly well accepted until the '70s. During this time, psychoanalysts Otto Kernburg and Heinz Kohut introduced the *narcissistic personality*, which they described as "exploitative and parasitic." Kohut would later go on to coin narcissistic personality disorder (NPD). He built on the theories that existed prior and ultimately used his discoveries to create his theory of self-psychology. In short, he believed that narcissistic people used their grandiose facade to hide insecurities, an idea that we still use when treating people with NPD.

Different psychologists eventually began looking at the different types and subtypes of narcissistic personality disorder to develop the classification system that we use today. Humanity has made a lot of progress in recognizing the depth of narcissism and everything that it entails, and there are still more studies being done as our world changes (George, 2018).

Megalomania

However, while the theories about narcissism began to rise in the late 19th century, another near-identical theory was developing at the same time: *megalomania*. A French neurologist coined this term to classify individuals who had fantasies of fame, power, self-aggrandizement, and other symptoms that we now recognize as a part of narcissistic personality disorder. People who had these traits were called megalomaniacs and were seen with fear and fascination by the people living in that time. The usage of the word spiked during World War II for predictable reasons, but it was eventually merged with NPD and is no longer even mentioned in the *Diagnostic and Statistical Manual of Mental Disorders (DSM)* as of 1980.

However, some people still insist that there is a slight difference between narcissism and megalomania, and they use the terms in different contexts. While narcissists are concerned with establishing superiority and making others believe that they are better than everyone else, a megalomaniac already sees themselves as superior and is only concerned with maintaining their reign. You can see how this term related to Adolf Hitler, the man to whom the term was most applied. Hitler already believed that Aryans were the superior race; he simply quested to give them the world—or, at least, that is what we are led to believe. If he had any internal doubts, he certainly did not display them in public.

However, despite these slight differences in terms, it is accurate to think of megalomania and narcissism as synonyms (or at least near-synonyms) in our modern age. You may see multiple professions use the word in tandem with narcissistic personality disorder, but do not let it confuse you. Nowadays, these words refer to the same disorder (Loudis, 2018).

Does My Sibling Know They Are a Narcissist?

Perceptions of normality will most likely be the factor to determine your sibling's awareness of their own narcissistic tendencies. Years of draining discomfort in your own experience may have been blissful from their point of view. The time they spend subjecting you to a sense of inferiority may have preserved their sense of superiority in return. The countless moments in which praise is won over or stolen may have made them used to special recognition while you have been deprived thereof.

Perhaps your graduation was overshadowed by an illness that was feigned in terms of its severity. Maybe their rebellious behaviors have garnered more concern than any committed effort of yours to be conscientious. It is possible that one small achievement of theirs appeared to trump your consistent stream of success in a diversity of things. In all these cases, patterns were shaped and then solidified. More than likely, these patterns resulted in your sibling shaping a perception that their behavior fell in the norm. They cannot recognize or even admit that the effects thereof have been damaging to one degree or another.

Has it ever occurred to you to ask your brother or sister outright whether they believe they are narcissistic? You may scoff at the very notion. Perhaps you can only imagine how such an attempt to label them would elicit their reactivity. They may see it as a challenge to their identity and would rather avoid the topic altogether. Or it is likely that you may find that they have never even considered the possibility.

However, you may be surprised to know that research has shown that self-report measures on narcissistic traits yielded more positive responses to the self-identification among people who actually scored high on personality inventories of narcissism (Psychology Today, 2019). That is significant, especially when you consider that if your narcissistic sibling was aware of these habits, they have made no motion toward taking stock or accountability for their actions.

In other words, even though some narcissists may recognize what they are, others remain blissfully ignorant. They are unaware simply because they haven't sat down and actually considered their behaviors objectively.

However, recent studies yield conflicting and even surprising results. Intuitively and even professionally, it has been long held that narcissists may not have known that their personality is detrimental to themselves or others. They have a personality structure that they find favorable, and their self-centeredness makes them incapable of recognizing its effects on others. Contrarily, some studies also discover that many do acknowledge the consequences of their entitlement and have evaluated the cost of their antisocial behaviors (Campbell & Crist, 2020).

There is also another consideration. Can your narcissistic sibling tell you that their behaviors are causing harm of some kind? When narcissistic traits border on dysfunctions that classify a psychological disorder, your sibling may actually be suffering from a condition that does not lie fully within their control.

Why Do People Develop Narcissistic Personality Disorder?

Perhaps one of the many prevailing questions in your mind is, why do narcissists exist in the first place? Rather, was your brother/sister born a narcissist, or were they unintentionally raised to become one?

It becomes a question of nature or nurture. "Nature" refers to the traits we are born with, and "nurture" refers to the traits inadvertently taught to us via our parents, peers, and the people around us. It is always difficult to distinguish between nature and nurture in any personality disorder, and NPD is no different. It can also vary from person to person, with some people being born with narcissistic traits and others becoming one over time. On average, experts credit inheritance to account for 60 percent of the traits, whereas the environment could be responsible for the remaining 40 percent (Keith & Crist, 2020).

Hereditary Factors

First among these deterministic factors is genetics. The complex arrangement of your sibling's DNA could thus be responsible for their inability to display empathy.

There has been a discovery of a recent gene called tryptophan hydroxylase-2 involved in regulating the production of the neurotransmitter serotonin, which is involved with a person's mood.

Research vouches that the possibility of developing narcissistic personality disorder increases if it is present in a person's family medical history (Paris, 2014). The impact of this factor is often studied in two ways: by investigating the genetic composition itself or by conducting twin studies (Burgemeester, 2020). The latter involves considering how identical twins, who share 100 percent of their genetic material, develop different personalities if raised by different families.

In other words, when you are examining your sibling, take a look at the other members of your family as well. Does anyone else display narcissistic tendencies, even if they display them in a different way? Has either of your parents mentioned struggling with empathy, self-esteem, or perfectionism in their youth? Examine your grandparents, aunts and uncles, and parents. Many people report having multiple narcissists in their families. Sometimes, multiple siblings all have narcissistic personality disorder, given that they have the same genetics and a similar upbringing. You may notice some interesting insights about your family when you pay attention to narcissistic tendencies.

Brain Structure

A second factor is added among the biological explanations for narcissism—brain structure. Through MRI scans, some studies have revealed that abnormalities in the density of a certain region on the cerebral cortex (the outer layer of the brain) may affect the individual's capacity for compassion (Schulze et al., 2013). This includes the way compassion is shaped and how it is processed when the person is exposed to it. The area called the left anterior insula was found to have less gray matter. Studies suggest that the volume of gray matter correlates with a person's ability to express empathy (Pedersen, 2013). Other studies confirm that a reduced brain volume in the prefrontal cortex is linked to the disorder (Nenadic et al., 2015). Still, more research is being done on how the brains of narcissists work. Future studies are set to reveal how regional exchanges within the brain further determine how short circuits in empathetic expression occur, as it is believed that a single location in the brain alone cannot be responsible.

Environmental Explanations

Perhaps the most evidence is found in the last factor, the narcissist's environment. Naturally, your immediate inclination is probably to view your family as the source of the problem. You think they allow your sibling's manipulations or do not notice them. However, about 10 percent of narcissism can be attributed to the family home. Parenting is the determining role player here. Grandiose narcissists grow up in households run by permissive parenting, where their transgressions of manipulations are allowed. In contrast, fragile narcissists are subjected to more hostile parenting styles. Thus, their manipulations seek to compensate instead of making others feed into their grandiosity (Keith & Crist, 2020).

Abuse, despite the abundant stereotypes, may occur in more than one form. Simple lessons that were perhaps envisioned to bestow a sense of strength and resilience on the child may have more effects than intended. Consider parents who believe that fueling their child's competitive spirit will make them successful and attempt to teach their children how to be "winners." Those parents may emphasize that winning yields recognition while losing leaves the child to become invisible. Also, think of the parent who indulges generously in their child's talents, breeding a belief that they are in many ways exceptional (Burgemeester, 2017).

The risk factors that stem from parental influence do not end there. Some children present their parents with needs that may be regarded as excessive and unnecessary, not warranting the degree of attention longed for. Similarly, their fears may be received with ridicule. Perhaps they are discounted or wholly unacknowledged. It could explain why these individuals engage in attention-seeking behaviors in later life, as a compensatory mechanism to counter the sense of emotional emptiness. Such parental responses may not form part of a consistent repertoire but instead manifest in a pattern of unreliable care. Alternatively, paternal responses could be predictable, either in the form of continuous criticism or excessive praise. Ultimately, it feeds into some of the most common signs of narcissism (i.e., lack of self-worth or an exaggerated belief therein).

Most of the time, though, narcissism develops outside of the shared environments. Understandably, your sibling is not exposed to parental influence through every moment of their lives. Their school, social circles, and leisure activities expose them to different influences altogether. This accounts for the range of personal experiences that contribute to narcissistic traits. Perhaps your brother befriends a group of physically deviant boys at school who engage in multiple antisocial behaviors that go unnoticed by any authority. Their ability to escape the consequences may have fed into their notions of power. Or maybe your sister fell in with a popular clique of girls. Because of her inclusion, she may have started to entertain ideas of superiority or special attention. There could be plenty of environmental factors at play here that you may or may not know about.

Whether through your parents or some other social or experiential sphere, many forms of narcissism stem from a sense of self-loathing. It could be that your sibling never is the bully but the victim of it. Perhaps they face many concealed incidents in which they question their self-worth. Trauma caused by emotional pain is a possible cause of narcissism.

However, despite our interpersonal networks, one cannot exclude a person's potential to fall prey to broader systems of influence. In this age of modernity, social media runs rampant to promote images of success. Hence, it is no wonder that we have grown ever more susceptible to a preoccupation with things like status, wealth, and appearance. Our online presence leads us to be more self-invested and crave more attention. For many technological migrants, the experience is relatively new. For anyone born as a late millennial and thereafter, it may have been all they have ever known. Though no conclusive research exists on the topic, we should not underestimate the impact of social conditioning. It leads us to question whether our obsession with ideal and virtual personas contributes to narcissistic personality traits.

Diathesis Stress Model

The best explanations for narcissism may not be tied to either predispositions or the environment exclusively but may instead be a result of the interplay between these forces. The *diathesis stress model* was first developed as a means of understanding depression and schizophrenia, but it has become a common way of understanding the development of many mental disorders in children and young adults (Li, 2020). It is a feasible explanation that attempts to lay out the trajectory of a disorder such as NPD. This model investigates how a predisposed susceptibility to the condition intersects with stressful life experiences (Abela & Hankin, 2005).

Your narcissistic sibling may likely have a stream of success in downplaying your problems in order to elevate theirs. Their purpose is perhaps to evoke pity (either in you or a family member) in order to shift blame away from themselves and maintain their image of being the tortured victim. According to the model, a biological predisposition (or diathesis) creates a possible susceptibility to develop NPD. When this interacts with a stress response, the disorder could be catalyzed. In your family, this stress may have manifested as a constant stream of belittling remarks flung at your sibling because of their perceived inadequacy in your parents' eyes. As the tally of derision adds up, eventually, the disorder develops, albeit in covert ways. The result is a self-absorption with their own shortcomings throughout their lives, leading them to seek fulfillment through dependency behaviors and calls for attention.

Of late, this model is used to determine the type of person at risk of developing psychopathology by looking into the interplay between genetic vulnerability (e.g., family's psychiatric history) and the stress level of a person (e.g., emotional trauma). The individual's level of resilience can determine their threshold to a certain amount of stress. If the individual's environmental stressors are below the threshold, nothing happens. Only when the pressure exceeds the individual's capability to bounce back that the disorder has a chance to develop (Lazarus, 1993).

In summary, even if an individual has a genetic predisposition to developing NPD, they still may not develop it unless their environment triggers it. Similar to how alcoholism is often inherited but can be easily avoided if an individual abstains from booze, someone who is at risk for NPD may not develop it if not for pressure from family, school, or any other part of the individual's life.

Why Am I Being Targeted?

Living with a narcissist can come with a lot of self-blame, doubt, and questioning. You may have been led to believe that you are ultimately at fault for your sibling's behavior, which may point you to a particular question: Why am I being targeted by my sibling?

Unfortunately, there is no straightforward answer to this. It is possible that by simply being their sibling, the narcissist has come to compare themselves to you or believes that others compare them to you. So naturally, they are determined to appear like they are "better" than you are, whether that means being smarter, more successful, or more physically attractive.

It is also possible that you have something that they want or are vulnerable in a way that makes you easy to target. As you read through the following lists, be sure to have an objective and self-accepting mindset. These lists are not intended to place the blame on you; they are simply meant to explain what a narcissist may be looking for so that you can better understand why you are the target of their manipulation and rage. We call these "green flags." Narcissists will pick up on these traits and take them as signals to begin abusing you.

- **Loneliness:** If you are isolated from the world, the narcissist will have an easier time abusing you in secret and turning people against you.
- **Financially stable:** Narcissists may target people who have a lot of money so that they can squander it for their personal endeavors.
- **Financially unstable:** On the flip side, if you need monetary support, a narcissist may use that as a way to make you dependent on them.
- **Being indecisive or lacking strong opinions:** If you do not hold strong morals or simply tend

to avoid confrontation, they may think you are less likely to stand up for yourself.

- **Low self-esteem:** People with low self-esteem are often more susceptible to compliments, making them easier to manipulate.
- **Having major fears:** If you have a major phobia or are fearful of the future, your sibling will likely provide comfort and make you dependent on them through that.
- **Childhood trauma:** The two of you probably shared a childhood, so your sibling may already be aware of certain traumas. Do they ever pretend to fix your issues, only to exploit your weaknesses later? If so, they are trying to create a dependency.
- **Compassion:** Being compassionate is a huge advantage in life, but it can be a disadvantage when you are dealing with a narcissist. They can use sad stories and personal traumas as a way to make you feel bad for them.
- **Intelligence:** In some cases, narcissists will target smart people and use them as a cover. If they were truly abusive, then how come this intelligent person has not seen through them? Alternatively, they may be jealous of your mind and try to make you take the backseat.
- **Responsibility:** If you take accountability for personal wrongdoings, a narcissist will try to

make you accountable for things you did not do and make you feel guilty.

As you can see, narcissists actually tend to target good people who will feel pity and empathy for them or those with insecurities that can be manipulated. In the long run, the things that you know will make you a better person might be the things that your sibling is taking advantage of, which is just another reason why the fault falls onto them, not you (Narcissist Abuse Support, 2019).

The WEB Method

Since you have already bought this book, you must have some evidence that is pointing you toward the conclusion that your sibling is a narcissist. You may even be thinking that it is highly likely, but unless you are a trained psychiatrist, you are probably having a few doubts. What if you are the one in the wrong? What if you are secretly harboring some jealousy or resentment against your sibling and this is how it is manifesting? What if you are incorrect and it is another disorder? These doubts may have come on your own, or your sibling may have planted them in your head already. To help alleviate these anxieties and give you a better idea of what to look for as you move forward with this book, I would like to introduce you to the WEB method. This method was invented by Bill Eddy, the author of *5 Types of People Who Can Ruin Your Life*, and it can give you a solid starting point as you are analyzing your relationship with your sibling. This method encourages you to look at three things: their words, your emotions, and their behavior.

Their Words

Actions speak louder than words, but we can all agree that words are still pretty loud. Even when softly spoken, words can manipulate, persuade, and tear relationships apart. They can also reveal hidden motives, which is particularly useful in the WEB method. Take a moment to recall some of your past interactions with your sibling, including the good and the bad. Think of some times that you have had fun with them, but also think of times that they have been hard to live with. If your sibling is a narcissist, you will likely notice one of these four patterns:

- **Extremely positive words:** Manipulation does not always mean put-downs and bullying. Oftentimes, it means flattery. It is good when someone compliments you and makes you feel good about yourself, so don't take every nice statement as a red flag. However, there are definitely some things you should look out for when your sibling talks to you. For starters, do their compliments usually involve some form of comparison? Does your sibling like to say "You are so much better than them," "Your last partner was a real loser," "You are better than this," or maybe "No one will know you better than I do"? Those types of compliments may be nice to hear sometimes, but they are often a signal that you will be negatively compared to others in the future as well.

- **Extremely negative words:** Again, most friendships and relationships with siblings involve some level of gossip and trash-talking, but take notice if your sibling has nothing good to say about anyone. Negative comments from a narcissist may also include some level of comparison and a sense of superiority, such as "I could do their job better than them," "He will be embarrassed when I am through with him," and similar statements. Even if someone legitimately screwed over your sibling, it is not healthy to engage in revenge fantasies. If they talk about others like that, imagine how they might talk about you.

- **Apathetic words:** A narcissist is unlikely to take an interest in your personal life. They have no real ability to relate to you, so they simply don't see the point in hearing how your day went or what you think about a certain topic. When you do try to talk about yourself, a narcissist may turn the conversation back to themselves. They may say, "Well, guess what happened to me!" or "That happened to me once," and then start telling an anecdote about their own lives. They might interrupt you when you speak, downplay your experiences, and show no excitement when you tell them about your achievements. There are a few exceptions, however. A narcissist might pretend to be interested until they feel they have earned your trust, so you may not see their true, apathetic nature until they feel like they have you trapped.

- **Victim words:** Does your sibling seem to go out of their way to convince you that they are the victim in every situation? Even if they were clearly in the wrong, do they find some way to twist the truth and convince everyone that they are an innocent victim? If so, you may be dealing with a narcissist. They struggle to see themselves as the bad guy in any situation, so they change the narrative until it fits with their self-image.

Your Emotions

When you are dealing with a potential narcissist, it is important not to discount your own feelings. It is always tempting to focus on the list of symptoms, be as objective as possible, and forget about the way your sibling makes you feel. However, your emotions can actually help you to discern the truth. Here's how:

- **Are you feeling too connected?** If someone is nice to you but rude to the waiter, they are not a good person. The same rule applies here: if your sibling acts out around everyone else but shows you their good side, it is possible that they are simply using you as a tool. They may purposefully try to make you dependent on them so that you can't leave, such as sabotaging your efforts to move out, be successful in school, and more. It may seem sweet that they don't want to lose you, but in reality, they are probably using you as a means to make themselves look better and don't want to have to find a new person for that. If you ever outshined them, they would be extremely upset with you.

- **Are you feeling stupid and having doubts?** Whether they do it on purpose or not, narcissists have a way of making us feel inadequate. It is a key aspect of the NPD gimmick to make others perceive themselves as worthless so that the narcissist can elevate their own image. You may even be feeling stupid for thinking your sibling is a narcissist since they project the idea that they are perfect in every way. Keep an eye out for these sorts of feelings in yourself as you continue reading.

- **Are you feeling suffocated?** Many people report feeling trapped when they are forced to interact with a narcissist. It is hard to get a word in, you can't talk about anything besides them, and you have to walk on eggshells to keep from offending them and inspiring yet another revenge plot. Being around your sibling might exhaust you and make you feel like you are gasping for breath.

Their Behavior

Even when a narcissist attempts to manipulate and charm, their actions will reveal their real motives. They will often try to hide their intentions and make themselves look innocent while they are pulling strings behind the scenes. Thus, you will have to have an investigative eye as you look back at past interactions. Here are some things to look for:

- **Disrespecting your wishes:** Communication is key in any relationship, especially when we are telling someone about our personal preferences and boundaries. In most relationships, communicating our boundaries is not a big deal so long as it is done politely. In fact, people in a healthy relationship will encourage that sort of conversation! This could not be further from the case for a narcissist, however. Even if you tell them your boundaries as politely and patiently as you possibly can, they will still get defensive or simply continue doing what you asked them not to. For instance, let us say your sibling has been borrowing your clothes without permission, which bothers you. You approach your sibling in private and tell them, "I don't mind if you want to borrow my clothes, but please let me know when you are going to do it so I don't plan on wearing it." A healthy individual would be understanding, but a narcissist would either lash out or be completely apathetic.

- **Projecting blame:** Since a narcissist refuses to recognize any personal faults, they look in other places when something goes wrong. If they do poorly on a test, they will blame you for distracting them. If they embarrass themselves at a job interview, they will blame you for snoring and keeping them up all night. Even if it is something small that does not have to be a big deal, they may be willing to make a scene just to prove that they did not do anything wrong. This includes situations they have made up, situations that they exaggerated, and situations that they have twisted the facts on.

Healthy people are willing to accept their flaws, even if it does sting at first, and will be willing to apologize if they falsely blamed you. A narcissist will not (Eddy, 2018).

Chapter 2:

Defining Narcissism

As many people know, the term "narcissism" comes from the Greek myth of Narcissus. Born of Cephissus (the personification of a Boeotian river) and a nymph, Narcissus was a handsome young man who broke the hearts of every girl he met. However, there was a catch: a seer warned his mother that Narcissus would only live a long life if he never "knew himself." Narcissus took extra precautions to avoid the prophecy until, one day, he looked at his reflection in a lake. Like so many young women (and a few men) before him, he fell in love. Naturally, Narcissus' reflection could not reciprocate the feeling. The poor boy pined there at the lakeside until he starved to death, as the seer foretold (Cartwright, 2017).

Ever since this myth became a part of Grecian life, Narcissus' name has become synonymous with arrogance and self-absorption. This is especially true if the person being labeled a narcissist is preoccupied with their looks. It is fairly common to label someone as a narcissist if they talk about themselves a lot or spend a long time looking in the mirror. Only about 1 percent of the population is diagnosed with NPD as a personality disorder. This number hasn't changed since the disorder was first recognized, even with the rise of social media and selfies, so it is clear that narcissism goes beyond caring about looks and fashion (Eddy, 2018). Unfortunately for psychologists, the myth of Narcissus has given people an inaccurate idea of everything that NPD encompasses.

Yes, many narcissists are obsessed with their looks, but it is not an encompassing symptom, and it does not appear in all types of NPD. Let us take a closer look at how psychologists define narcissism and its various types and subtypes.

Understanding Narcissism

Personality Disorders vs. Mental Illnesses

NPD stands for narcissistic personality disorder. What exactly is a personality disorder, and how does it differ from mental illness? Well, it is a little complicated. Let us start by looking all the way back to Germany in the 1890s.

Koch, a German psychiatrist, noticed that there was a milder form of mental illness among a number of his patients, so he coined the term "psychopathic" to describe these cases. According to him, "even in bad cases, the irregularities do not amount to mental illness"

(Kendell, 2018). During Koch's time, the only "mental illnesses" that were recognized were insanity and idiocy. Understandably, he began noticing certain individuals who didn't suit either of these faulty labels. As more and more mental illnesses were discovered, the "mild" disorders that Koch and some of his colleagues noticed became known as personality disorders.

To this day, there is debate over whether or not personality disorders should be considered a mental illness. Kurt Schneider, another German psychiatrist, has stated that personality disorders are "abnormal varieties of sane psychic life." He means that people with personality disorders simply see the world differently and don't require any treatment. Many European countries have maintained this view, but others see personality disorders as a subset of mental illness that can often be very serious (Kendell, 2018).

Regardless of how psychiatrists choose to view personality disorders, they all agree on how they should be classified and what makes them different from mental illness. The International Classification of Mental and Behavioral Disorders (ICD-10) explains that personality disorders are unique because they are "deeply ingrained and enduring behavior patterns, manifesting themselves as inflexible responses to a broad range of personal and social situations" that appear in childhood and remain for the majority of the patient's life, especially if left untreated (Kendell, 2018). They are long-lasting, persistent, and affect an individual's basic thought processes, which often allows them to change every decision a person makes.

According to Robitz (2o18), modern psychology recognizes 10 personality disorders:

1. Antisocial personality disorder
2. Avoidant personality disorder
3. Borderline personality disorder
4. Dependent personality disorder
5. Obsessive-compulsive personality disorder
6. Paranoid personality disorder
7. Histrionic personality disorder
8. Schizoid personality disorder
9. Schizotypal personality disorder
10. Narcissistic personality disorder

People with one of these 10 personality disorders are at a higher risk for mental illnesses, such as depression and anxiety. They also are more likely to engage in substance abuse and self-harm. The presence of a personality disorder on top of mental illness also makes treatment a lot more complicated. The individual may not bond as readily with their therapist. They may be more likely to lie about their symptoms and interrupt other patients' progress in a group therapy session. Also, the personality disorder's outward symptoms may make it harder to find a clear diagnosis for the mental illness. Because of this, most psychiatrists consider personality disorders an important complication, if not a mental illness in its own right (Kendell, 2018).

DSM-5 Criteria

DSM-5 is short for *Diagnostic and Statistical Manual of Mental Disorders, 5th Edition*. It is a book by the American Psychiatric Association that is used as the end-all-be-all for defining mental disorders. This book helps psychiatrists around the country give consistent diagnoses when dealing with mental disorders and personality disorders, which are often quite subjective in nature. If you are looking for a concrete definition of NPD, the DSM-5 is the place to go!

Here are the criteria for a person to be diagnosed with a narcissistic personality disorder, according to the American Psychiatric Association (2013):

- Having an inflated sense of self-importance and entitlement
- Needing constant admiration and praise
- Expecting special treatment due to perceived superiority
- Exaggerating achievements and talents
- Reacting negatively to criticism
- Being preoccupied with fantasies about power, success, and beauty
- Taking advantage of others
- Having an inability or unwillingness to recognize the needs and feelings of other people
- Behaving in an arrogant manner

Although the DSM-5 can be used as a useful guide in recognizing NPD, it only lists the most common symptoms and sometimes neglects the more allusive aspects of the disorder. For instance, many narcissists experience feelings of emptiness and boredom alongside the traits listed above. They find that the world does not fulfill them and therefore struggle to apply themselves to a particular career or goal. Not all narcissists are well-dressed and successful; many are seen as slackers for this exact reason (Caligor, 2015). In general, the DSM-5 can be used as a guideline, but the exact nature of your sibling's narcissism may vary. We will explore some more variations in a bit.

Diagnosing and Treating Narcissistic Personality Disorder

Narcissists are infamously resistant to going to therapy. Most types think they are perfect in every way, so what could a therapist possibly help them with? However, in some cases, a person with NPD who also struggles with substance abuse or another diagnosable illness will begin attending therapy for the secondary issue. Then the therapist will notice the underlying personality disorder. From the moment the therapist sees narcissistic tendencies, they must tread very carefully if they don't want to upset their client and risk having them shut down.

In order to diagnose a narcissist, the client must fulfill the following criteria:

- **Impairments when perceiving their identity:** A narcissist will have an exaggeratedly positive view of their own performance in life, or they may fluctuate between extreme confidence and extreme anxiety. They may also obsess over other people's opinions, have perfectionistic views, or feel so entitled to a good life that they struggle to motivate themselves to chase after things they really want. They would rather have their dreams delivered at their doorstep.
- **Impairments in interpersonal relations:** Since narcissists struggle to care about others, looking at a person's intimate relationships is a good way to tell whether they are a narcissist. Someone with NPD will only care about others' problems if it starts to affect them personally, which causes a lot of turmoil in all of their relationships. Most of the time, their friendships and romances only last for a short while.
- **Possession of pathological personality traits:** This requirement essentially means that the individual must meet all the symptoms listed in the DSM-5, which we looked at earlier. Taking the time to examine these symptoms will help a psychiatrist be certain that the patient has NPD and not any of the other nine personality disorders.

- **Consistency of symptoms over a long period with no other probable causes:** If someone is having a bad week (or even a bad month!), they might show some or all of these symptoms. However, a true narcissist will possess these traits for all of their adult life, so it is important to examine whether these tendencies are a pattern or just a temporary mood. The psychiatrist should also be able to rule out other possibilities, such as similar personality disorders.

Once a diagnosis is made, the patient can begin looking at treatment. We will look closer at specific therapeutic treatments for NPD in a later chapter in more detail, but I will provide a quick summary to give you an idea of what we are dealing with. Although medication exists to treat mental illness, such as depression, anxiety, and ADHD, personality disorders do not react to any medication that modern science is aware of. If a narcissist is put on medication, it will be to lessen the symptoms of a coexisting condition. Since medicine is not an option, the patient will be directed to therapy instead. Individual, group, and family therapy can all be effective treatments for NPD, especially if they are pursued in the long term.

Cognitive behavioral therapy is a favorite of the modern therapist. It can be used to redirect a narcissist's distorted thoughts with something more realistic but still ultimately positive in nature. Through psychodynamic therapy, the therapist and patient will work together to examine the narcissist's past to determine the root cause of the problematic ideas. If the narcissist is still living with you, your parents, or another guardian, family therapy will probably be offered. NPD affects the whole family, so a therapist will be interested in hearing from each person in the household.

Ultimately, the aim is to redirect the narcissist's thoughts. Although it is tempting to try taking their ego down a peg to balance out their arrogant ideas, doing so will often have the opposite effect as the narcissist becomes defensive or finds their shaky self-esteem is even more challenged. The key is to understand that their perception of the world is warped, so the treatment is only effective if their ability to navigate reality is corrected. They should not be told that they are actually below average; they should be told that everyone is equal and that that is okay.

If your sibling can't be convinced to go to therapy, have no worries. It is not your responsibility to "fix" them, and being too persistent can put you in a dangerous position. This book will teach you how to live peacefully with a narcissist, not how to correct their behavior on your own.

The "False Self"

With all this talk of how narcissists see the world through distorted vision, you may be curious to understand exactly what your sibling sees. It is hard to imagine being purposefully cruel, especially when you know that everyone has reasons behind their actions. You may find it helpful to think about the *false self* when you are interacting with your sibling to help you understand them a little bit better.

The false self has to do with the facade that your sibling puts forward. You know the one: the fake personality that they hide behind in public settings. It is the act they put on in front of your parents and the cute little voice they use to get everything they want. They seem to be capable of molding their personality according to whatever they think their audience will respond to the most. Hence, unless you know them very well, it is difficult to determine what their true personality is.

Narcissists often dissociate (that is, disconnect from themselves) when they enter their "false self" state. They may feel absent from their bodies during the duration. It is as though they are controlling a video game character instead of operating their body in the real world. That is how their act is so convincing. They take a step back from the controls and allow their false self to take the wheel. It is likely they are being possessed by an alter ego. In some cases, this is the self that the narcissistic idealizes and glorifies. Since their false self performs so well in front of others, they believe that they are superior to everyone else and begin to behave as though they are. This is especially the case in narcissists who are more manipulative since they use their false self to deceive the people around them.

Unfortunately for the narcissist, dissociating and slipping into their false self can have a major consequence: memory failure. When they are so disconnected from their true self, they have a hard time fully processing the things that happen to them. Conversations start to blend together. The exact details of events slip under the rug, and things like time and location become unclear. The nature of NPD may also lead their minds to forget details that challenge their idea of superiority. Your narcissistic sibling has not chosen to ignore their obvious faults; they have forgotten about them entirely!

Believe it or not, this cycle of dissociating and forgetting is the direct cause of their habitual lying. Psychiatrists call this "confabulation," or the act of making assumptions about an event when the exact details have been forgotten. We all confabulate a little bit in our lives, especially when it comes to our early childhood, but narcissists do it constantly. They don't remember everything that happened when they were dissociating, so their minds make assumptions about how things must have gone. Sam Vaknin, Professor of Psychology at South Federal University, words it best: "They invent plausible 'plugins' and scenarios of how things might, could, or should have plausibly occurred. To outsiders, these fictional stopgaps appear as lies. But the narcissist fervently believes in their reality: He may not actually remember what had happened, but surely it could not have happened any other way" (Vaknin, 2020).

In other words, the narcissist's reality is warped from their constant dissociation. Even if they don't mean to tell lies, they end up speaking untruths anyway because their minds have fabricated a lot of the things that have happened to them. When your narcissistic brother exaggerates how awful you are to him when you simply criticize his tone of voice, he likely believes that you are, indeed, that awful to him. Likewise, if your narcissistic older sister says that everyone at the party loves her when they actually find her absolutely obnoxious, her mind has probably invented that reality all on its own.

Why Does the False Self Exist?

Understandably, you may find yourself a bit frustrated at the existence of the false self in the first place. Is it so hard to be yourself in public? Why put up a front all of the time? Although your frustrations are extremely reasonable, it is often not as simple as just "being yourself."

As Vaknin explains, the false self exists for two main purposes. The first is that the narcissist believes their true self to be their false self. When you believe that your sibling is being fake and superficial, they think that they are being their best selves at that moment, and this is what gives them their superiority complex. Their false self can be extremely charming and socially adept, so they think that they deserve praise for this behavior. For this reason, separating the narcissist from their false self is extremely difficult. Secondly, the false self exists as a defense mechanism. Dissociating from reality and forgetting about life events is an easy way to escape trauma, pain, anxiety, and depression. It is as though the narcissist has escaped into a fantasy where they are the king or queen and the rest of the world does not have to matter. When the narcissist does engage with reality, it is only when they are treated the way they want to be treated (Vaknin, 2020).

Triangulation

Triangulation is a phenomenon that exists in multiple social dynamics, but it is particularly common when a narcissist is involved. Triangulation occurs when a third person is brought into a relationship as a means of comparison. The third person is used to threaten the original pairing with the possibility of being replaced, removed from the triangle, or simply made to feel that they are somehow "lesser" than the new member of the triangle.

Here is an example. Sara and Cindy are two young sisters, and Cindy, the older one, is a narcissist. Cindy is typically nice to Sara when the two of them are alone, but when Cindy's friend Ann is around, Cindy pits Ann and Sara against each other and shows a major preference for Ann. Sara is left feeling like she needs to fight for Cindy's attention and thinking she is not as important as Ann.

Triangulation helps feed a narcissist's ego because it portrays Cindy as a prize that Sara has to fight for, and it makes Cindy feel very important and desirable. It also makes Cindy feel more secure in her relationships, as both Sara and Ann will be dependent on her. Sara will be fighting for attention, and Ann will be desperate to maintain her position as the "favorite." Cindy has a lot of power in this dynamic.

If your sibling ever triangulates, it may be a sign of their manipulative nature and desire to be seen as superior. Take notice of that sort of behavior and distance yourself when it happens; it is not beneficial to anyone who is a part of the triangle (Greenberg, 2020).

Comorbidities and Other Complications

If you have a narcissistic sibling, you may already be aware of some common comorbidities. Comorbidities are diseases that exist simultaneously in the same individual, and they can be extremely common with mental illness and personality disorders. For instance, many individuals who suffer from depression will also have anxiety, and it can be difficult to separate the two diseases since some symptoms can overlap and exacerbate each other.

NPD also has an extremely high rate of comorbidities. A study performed by a group of psychiatrists in 2008 revealed some interesting statistics about narcissists in America and how the disorder typically affects different genders.

As the study discovered, comorbidities are slightly more common in male narcissists than females. However, both are at extremely high risk for substance abuse of all kinds. According to Stinson (2008), they can be up to 18.5% more likely to be dependent on alcohol, 24.1% more likely to be addicted to drugs, and 11.6% more likely to have a nicotine addiction. Narcissists are also extremely likely to have a secondary mood disorder, with the most common ones being major depressive disorder (10.4%), bipolar disorder (31.1%), generalized anxiety (22.1%), and posttraumatic stress disorder (18.6%). They are also likely to suffer from panic disorder with agoraphobia. That is, they fear situations that may cause embarrassment or helplessness. They have a 23.9% chance of suffering from this phobia, which makes sense because those sorts of situations would challenge their self-image.

However, although narcissists are slightly more prone to depression, they typically do not struggle with suicidal thoughts. Why would the majority of narcissists avoid this single symptom? As Vaknin (2020) explains, "The simple answer is that they died a long time ago. Narcissists are the true zombies of the world." Because they exist as their false selves in the majority of their interactions, they have already effectively erased their true personalities and become the person they would rather be. When a therapist is working with a patient who has both NPD and depression, they typically build a new, healthier self rather than trying to revive the remnants of the true self. The true self will be too far gone to recover, but it can be built back up with new traits, habits, and tendencies. However, if the narcissist's true self is still observable, then it can be recovered in some sense through intensive therapy (Vaknin, 2020).

Self-Absorption vs. Narcissism

The difference between someone who is obsessed with their looks and someone who has NPD is the amount in which the disorder interferes with their lifestyle. This is regardless of whether their symptoms are occasional or constant and whether or not they are simply hiding their insecurities.

First of all, take a look at how much their symptoms have taken over your sibling's daily life. Your aunt Kate may be overly concerned about her weight, and her diet may be a little bit unhealthy. However, she is not a true narcissist unless her goals have begun to ruin her relationships, become more important than her hobbies, and taken over her life. In fact, most narcissists struggle to fall in love because they do not find commitment very exciting: they are more interested in the flirting stages of a relationship when their partner pays them lots of compliments. This makes them more likely to pursue hook-ups and one-night-stands than the average person. As you can see, NPD will affect all parts of a narcissist's life, including their romantic endeavors. Remember that personality disorders are long-lasting, and they change an individual's thought patterns. Hence, it makes sense that their disorder will cloud their overall judgment.

Most people assume one of two things about a narcissist: They either think that a narcissist has an overabundance of self-confidence, or they assume that a narcissist is secretly self-conscious, which is why they desire so much praise and attention. Neither of these assumptions is fully correct. In truth, a narcissist craves appreciation and admiration, and they want to be seen as better than their peers. Self-esteem issues could potentially be related to this desire, but they don't have to be. A narcissist is different from a normal person who likes compliments as they are a little bit too self-critical.

Also, most people who have NPD will constantly be rude and demeaning to others. We all have bad days and occasionally say things that may be deemed inappropriate, but a narcissist is mean all of the time. It is a part of their core personality rather than a sign that they are having a bad day. This is related to the narcissist's apathy. They don't really care about the people around them, so they see no harm in spewing insults. They also will not care about your personal accomplishments and achievements, unlike someone who is a little insecure.

To tell the difference between someone who is self-absorbed or self-conscious and someone who has NPD, ask yourself the following questions:

- Does this person struggle to show humility?
- Does this person get defensive in the face of criticism, no matter what part of themselves is being criticized?
- Does this person appear to have no insecurities?
- Is this person consistently unpleasant to be around?
- Has rudeness become a pattern?
- Does this person dismiss my achievements?
- Do they appear uncaring when I tell them that I have completed a goal of my own?

If you answer yes to these questions when you think about your sibling, then your sibling is a narcissist rather than someone who is preoccupied with their appearance or any other insecurity.

Types of Narcissistic Personality Disorder

Many mental disorders have different types that can help us recognize the specifics of the symptoms. Even depression, a common disorder, is an umbrella term. A person may have major depression, seasonal depression, postpartum depression, and many more. In the same sense, psychiatrists recognize a number of types and subtypes of NPD that help to quantify the specific behaviors of a client. As you read about the following categories, think about your sibling and try to identify which heading they might fit under.

Classic Narcissists

Kate is the oldest sister of three, and she paved the way for her siblings. She was the first to enter high school, the first to graduate college, and the first to get an impressive position at a law firm. She is quick to talk about her achievements to others, and when her words are not flaunting her wealth, her clothes are. She is a skilled socialite and an undeniable beauty, and she gets whatever she wants. Many of her peers from school admire her, but those who are close to her know that something is amiss. Kate is a narcissist. She is unwilling to talk about anyone else's life, and she struggles with empathy ever since she was young. If her siblings or parents try to convince her to work on herself, she gets aggressive and insists that nothing is wrong.

Had Kate gone to a psychiatrist, she would have learned that she is a classic narcissist. You may also see this form of narcissism referred to as high-functioning or grandiose. This is the type we have been talking about the most so far in this book, and it is what most people think of when they imagine a narcissist: an attention-seeking braggart who gets bored when someone else takes the spotlight. They see themselves as superior, and they need everyone around them to agree.

The name "high-functioning" comes from the fact that these narcissists are usually very successful and sometimes don't encounter any tremendous downfalls because of their disorders. They may be seen as effective leaders, bosses, politicians, and plenty more. Even if they come across as arrogant, they are often very difficult to diagnose because they simply seem like a person with an abundance of confidence. These types are usually very extroverted and charming, and they often seek special treatment.

However, apathy is where they differ from neurotypical people. A classic narcissist is unafraid to ruin relationships in order to get the spotlight back on themselves. They struggle to show empathy for others, and they sabotage others with no regrets.

Vulnerable Narcissists

Joey is the youngest sibling of his family, and his older brother John knows he is a narcissist. Everyone else seems oblivious. Joey is quiet, polite, and sometimes generous to a fault. He gives until he gets himself in trouble, which some see as a simple lack of boundaries. However, John knows that his little brother engages in a deep-seated messiah complex and loves being complimented for his self-sacrificing behavior. When he tries to point this out to anyone, he is labeled jealous or rude. Joey also likes to complain excessively about minor offenses. He tells white lies about how hard his life is and almost begs for pity. He needs the world to see him as a tortured soul, and he does it through manipulative means.

Vulnerable narcissists like Joey are also called compensatory, closet, or fragile. Their personalities vary quite drastically from the classic narcissist. Although they still feel superior and want to be treated accordingly, they don't like the spotlight. They may be introverted and insecure, or they simply lack the social prowess of the classic narcissist. Because of this, they seek the attention they are looking for in other ways.

Many people under this type seek pity rather than outright attention. They may paint themselves as a constant victim. They exaggerate negative feelings or even downright lie about their personal traumas and experiences to convince the people around them to feel bad for them. On the opposite end of the spectrum, vulnerable narcissists may use excessive kindness or self-sacrifice in order to seek the praise of the people they are aiming to help. Showing kindness makes everyone feel good, but this type of NPD takes it to another level.

Earlier, I mentioned that a number of narcissists do experience low self-esteem. This type contains the majority of those individuals. If your sibling wants others to elevate them while also hating themselves, they may fall into this category.

Malignant Narcissists

Tom is Greta's older brother, and he is moving out to attend the college of his dreams. Greta's parents celebrate his success, but Greta celebrates no longer having to see him every day. For Greta, growing up under the same roof as Tom is traumatizing. All older brothers can be bullies sometimes, but Tom takes an unusual amount of pleasure in tormenting Greta in front of her parents and even her friends. Worst of all, he successfully convinces their parents that he is the victim! Thankfully, now that Tom's going to college, Greta will have to endure less of his scheming, manipulating, and lying.

Malignant narcissists like Tom are also called toxic narcissists—and for a good reason. Their arrogance displays itself as a general hatred for other people. They are often antisocial, manipulative, and passive-aggressive. They are likely to engage in revenge plots when things don't go their way. When others do not recognize their self-perceived superiority, they believe the other party is at fault for not seeing what they think is common sense.

In a lot of cases, malignant narcissists will also fulfill the requirements needed to be diagnosed as a sociopath or psychopath, so you may see some similarity between those behaviors. Many take pleasure in being ruthless toward others. They are chronic liars and enjoy intimidating the people around them.

This type is the most difficult for therapists to work with because they usually exhibit the same behavior to the people trying to help them. They may lie their way out of treatment, frighten or threaten their therapist, or seek revenge if the therapist attempts to criticize their narcissistic traits.

Subtypes of Narcissistic Personality Disorder

Alongside the three main types of NPD, a narcissist may also exhibit traits of a number of subtypes: overt, covert, somatic, or cerebral. The subtypes all describe very specific behaviors that a narcissist may exhibit. They help to describe the exact nature of the narcissist, how they see themselves, and how they approach the world. The types and subtypes typically overlap such that everyone in the three main types will also show tendencies toward the subtypes in some way.

Overt vs. Covert

Whether a narcissist is overt or covert will be determined by how subtle they are about getting the attention they desire. The overt narcissist will be pretty upfront. They are vocal about their intentions, their actions are clearly self-centered, and they go out of their way to put people down. Kate, the older sister from our example earlier, is an overt narcissist. In fact, all classic narcissists will be overt as a part of the diagnosis.

Joey, the little brother from earlier, is covert. Although he is definitely a narcissist, his methods are more secretive. He prefers to work behind the scenes. He lies, manipulates, and attempts to gain people's trust in order to get what he wants. Joey is also a little more difficult to diagnose since his narcissistic tendencies are harder to see. However, he is also dangerous in own way because he is more manipulative than his overt counterparts.

Malignant narcissists like Tom can go either way. Tom himself is more covert since he deceives others into thinking that he is the better sibling and Greta is the bad guy. However, there are plenty of malignant narcissists who are more overt. Those individuals are often outwardly pushy and confrontational. They will take any opportunity they see to brag about themselves. They are usually not as charming as characters like Tom and have a hard time integrating with normal life.

Somatic vs. Cerebral

This subtype is used to label what the narcissist cares about in themselves and others. This is typically what they believe makes them superior (or, in the case of the vulnerable narcissist, what makes them secretly insecure). It is possible for a narcissist to value both of these subtypes, but they typically prioritize one over the other in a notable way. If it is too hard to choose one over the other, don't worry about it! It is not necessary for the diagnosis.

The majority of the narcissists I used in my examples are cerebral in nature. This means that they believe they are intellectually or morally superior to everyone else. These are the narcissists who brag about their grades, career, recent placement on the student board, and anything that proves they are smarter than you. They may also go out of their way to make themselves look like a better person than you, even if they have to sabotage your reputation in order to make it happen.

However, if a narcissist is somatic, they care more about their looks and body. They are often obsessed with looking young. Hence, they spend a lot of time at the gym and absolutely love posting selfies. They buy a lot of personal bling, modify their body, or switch up their hairstyle every month. They would never date someone who is more attractive than them because they don't want to be outshined, and they certainly want to be regarded as the "pretty sibling" as well. If they don't feel like the prettiest in the room, they may try to sabotage others so that they can earn the spot for themselves. Narcissus from the Greek myth is certainly a somatic narcissist, and Kate displays a few characteristics of this subtype as well.

Unlike with overt and covert subtypes, any narcissist from any of the main three types can be either cerebral or somatic. This subtype has less to do with how they display symptoms and more to do with what their mind is obsessed with. Hence, it is possible for any narcissist to fall into either side of the spectrum.

Chapter 3:

Breaking Down Narcissism

Now that we have taken an in-depth look at the nature of narcissism and why it causes your sibling to act the way they do, let us zoom in on the different types of narcissism and see how they function. In this chapter, you will receive more examples of each type so that you can grow more familiar with narcissistic behavior. We will also tackle how these behaviors can manifest and how to categorize them into the different types and subtypes you are already familiar with. You may notice a lot of familiar situations, but you will also see types of narcissism that you have not yet been exposed to, so having a broader range of knowledge will help you recognize the exact brand of narcissism that your sibling falls under.

At the end of each example, I will give a short analysis of each narcissist and explain why I believe they fall into the category I have sorted them into. Since I don't know these individuals in real life, I can't give a complete diagnosis, but I will examine their behaviors as they have been described and give my thoughts. I will also mention some of the topics we have covered thus far, such as the false self and comorbidities.

Classic Narcissists

From the last chapter, you will remember that classic narcissists are the type that most people think of when they try to imagine a narcissist. They are charming, often extroverted, and quick to brag. They are exclusively overt in nature—meaning, their methods are straightforward and upfront rather than manipulative. Since their symptoms are so visible and easily fit into the stereotypes of a narcissist, they are also extremely easy to diagnose in most cases. The people around them can recognize their self-centered ways, even if they can't do anything about it or fall under the narcissist's charm.

Living with a classic narcissist can be particularly frustrating because they tend to be successful and can often climb to the top with ease and grace. However, if you know the narcissist, you know the true story. They step on other people and are willing to treat others unfairly. Also, they often take credit for things they have not done in order to get ahead. The outside world may see them as an effective businessperson, but they are actually megalomaniacs.

However, their success in their careers has an ultimate downfall: they are extremely poor at decision-making. Research has shown that narcissists, particularly classic narcissists, are prone to impulse decisions because they cannot see the negatives of a situation. For instance, if a classic narcissist is leading a business and is given an offer with a setback as high as 30 percent, they are more likely to take that deal compared to someone with normal self-esteem. They see themselves as above the statistics and can't imagine themselves failing at anything, so they see no harm in taking major risks. Research in finance has shown that narcissistic CEOs are more likely to engage in shady, illegal practices and commit fraud, but they don't see much success in taking shortcuts. In fact, their businesses "more likely have volatile stock prices but not perform better in financial terms. They are more likely to engage in more acquisitions and to overpay for these" (O'Reilly, 2021).

Later on, we will look at how a narcissist's brain structure leads them to make brash decisions. For now, let us examine two real-life examples of classic narcissists and see how they attempt to manipulate and cheat their way into the spotlight.

Example 1: The Fake Miscarriage

Reddit user Former_Trainer6705 shared the situation her family dealt with because of her narcissistic sister. She is one of three sisters—the eldest, the narcissist, and herself. The narcissistic sister "only loves three things: money, attention, and sympathy." She has been a problem child since she was young, but things escalated when their eldest sister had a miscarriage.

Understandably, the family was in mourning. The eldest sister had been wanting a child and was absolutely devastated when she received news of the miscarriage. The family was ready to support her. For the next week, she received loads of well-earned love and attention. Unfortunately, however, a narcissist hates when anyone else has the spotlight, even in times of grief.

While the family was still in mourning, the narcissist called a family meeting and summoned her best crocodile tears. Through her sobs, she told the family that she, just like her eldest sibling, had become pregnant and lost her child. The Reddit poster explains that this is nigh-impossible thanks to a medical condition the narcissist has that makes her essentially infertile. Understandably, the eldest sibling was upset by the lie and blew up in anger as she accused the narcissistic sister of lying. Their relationship never recovered. Later, the family would find three pregnancy tests in the bathroom garbage bin. All three read negative, solidifying their evidence that the narcissist had lied in order to steal attention from her grieving sister. However, as the poster tells us, she faced no consequences for her actions because their parents struggle to stand up to her.

Although it is impossible to give a complete diagnosis through one situation alone, the behavior seen here is typical of a classic narcissist. Her methods were extremely overt, especially the concept of orchestrating an entire family meeting just to announce a lie. Only caring about money, attention, and sympathy also speaks of a classic narcissist since they tend to value their social success a little more than other types. This narcissist seems to struggle deeply with her false self.

Through dissociation and confabulation, she might have constructed the idea that she had a miscarriage in her mind and felt confident enough in that reality to act upon it.

Example 2: The Tough Lover

This story was shared on Reddit by a deleted user named Alice. Alice is the oldest of five siblings, and the youngest three were born with mental disabilities, so they required a bit of extra help. This was especially true when their mother passed away. Alice, as the oldest sibling, took on the responsibility of helping her youngest siblings grow more independent in spite of their disabilities. The second oldest sibling, Laura, was living with her boyfriend at the time, but she would stop by on occasion to "help" Alice raise their younger siblings. Laura was also a classic narcissist.

Laura liked to point out that Alice was "incapable" of taking care of their younger siblings and the household, so she would take matters into her own hands. Laura would constantly point out everyone's shortcomings and call it "tough love" if any of them disagreed with her methods. She thought Alice was too soft on their siblings, so she decided it was best to make them feel miserable and stupid when they failed to perform certain tasks, such as filling out job applications. The family's relationship with Laura got worse and worse until Alice came to a realization: Laura never really cared about the family; "it was always about how she

71

appeared in front of everyone else." As a narcissist, Laura put down her siblings in order to make herself look and feel superior, so her guise of "tough love" was actually just an excuse to bully her siblings. The siblings have cut off contact with Laura and have lived a better life ever since.

Laura seems to display the behavior of a classic narcissist. She is a proud antagonizer, constantly puts down others, and takes any opportunity she can to put herself above Alice and her other siblings. Her excuse of "tough love" may be a manipulation tactic, a means of denying her behavior, or simply a means of elevating herself since she seemed to think tough love was the best means of raising her siblings. Her tactics are very overt, seen in the way she insulted others to their face and asserted that her techniques were better.

Vulnerable Narcissists

As we covered in the last chapter, vulnerable narcissists are the sneakiest form of NPD. They are more manipulative, are more likely to lie and play the victim, and use more passive-aggressive means to make themselves feel superior. They are always covert— meaning, they act behind the scenes to try to change people's feelings toward them. They can be a bit harder to diagnose, especially since they are more likely to have comorbid disorders. However, those who are closest to them can see that they are obsessed with their self-image. Unfortunately, however, they often fool others into thinking that they are the victim in every situation and can, therefore, ostracize an individual and turn the world against them.

If you are having some trouble distinguishing whether your sibling is a classic or vulnerable narcissist, think back to a moment when someone criticized your sibling. It could be a big or small criticism—it does not matter. Maybe your parents tried to call them out on not completing a chore. Maybe one of their peers at school gave them an honest critique on an assignment they did not put their best into. Or maybe it was the last time that you fought with them and threw some insults around. Either way, your narcissist sibling likely responded in one of two ways: complete and utter dismissal or absolute offense (maybe even a breakdown).

If your sibling dismissed the criticism and seemed unworried about it, they are probably a classic narcissist. That type is more secure with themselves, so they likely believe that anything said against them is inaccurate. They might even tie in a bit of gaslighting and try to convince you that you are the crazy one for insisting they have any flaws. The vulnerable narcissist, however, will get defensive. They are more neurotic than their classic counterparts—meaning, they have a higher tendency toward anxiety, insecurity, and self-doubt. They likely try to hide these feelings behind a kind and generous facade, but they are secretly struggling with a lot of negative emotions.

A vulnerable narcissist may also bear more similarities with borderline personality disorder. BPD is marked by extreme emotions that often swing from one end of the spectrum to another. They may adore their friends one day but decide they absolutely hate them if there is any drama between them. People with BPD also have a flawed perception of self and very low self-esteem. They resort to escapism or self-harm to cope with negative feelings, and they are likely to have depression, anxiety, and suicidal thoughts. In fact, I find it helpful to think of a vulnerable narcissist as someone with BPD who is also manipulative and hides behind a mask.

If you are still struggling to categorize your sibling, the following real-life examples may help. One is an insecure sister who shows strong, vulnerable characteristics, and another is a diagnosed narcissist who is willing to share his story to help others.

Example 1: The Copycat Sister

One poster on Beyondblue.org shared her story about her sister back in January of 2016. She opened her post with the following: "Yet again, I have left my mum's house in tears. My sister is a complete narcissist and has my mum completely under her spell." Her sister has been telling lies to their mother in the hopes of making her feel guilty and placing the blame anywhere but her. The narcissist likes to whisper in their mom's ear even when her sister is around to visit, which causes frequent fights that only end in misplaced blame and hurt feelings. "She has accused me of being jealous of her and not supporting her, and I am sick of being there when she won't help herself."

Although the poster wishes she could simply stop seeing her sister, creating distance is hard when the sister still lives with their mom, with whom the poster has a close relationship and tries to visit frequently. Unfortunately, she nearly lost her mom's trust thanks to the narcissist's constant lies.

Interestingly, although the narcissist likes to claim that the poster is jealous of her, the narcissist displays some jealousy of her own as well. She got married nine months after her sister did, moved into a house near one that her sister nearly bought, and seems to follow her sister wherever she goes. Like many narcissists, it seems that she does not want to lose the one person she uses as a scapegoat in order to elevate herself. It is also possible that she is secretly very insecure, so she copies her sister in order to feel successful and to avoid feeling like her sister "won."

Because of these hints at insecurity and her covert methods of manipulation, it seems clear that this narcissist falls under the vulnerable category. She desires pity and wants to be seen as the victim in everything, which is especially common in this type. She is not upfront enough to be the classic type, but she also is not aggressive enough to be malignant, so this seems like the proper placement for her.

Example 2: The Recovering Narcissist

Since vulnerable narcissists are harder to diagnose and understand, let us take a look at a diagnosed vulnerable narcissist and see what he has to say. Reddit user Casualiama shared a post explaining his diagnosis and invited others to ask him anything.

Casualiama says that he received his diagnosis about a year after he researched vulnerable narcissism. After the diagnosis, he felt extremely depressed and ashamed and believed that no amount of treatment was going to help him. Thankfully, however, he has made a lot of progress since that point, and no longer does he feel so hopeless. His symptoms have lessened, his relationships have improved, and he has a more realistic outlook on life.

However, before Casualiama began recovering, he was obsessed with compliments, social recognition, and making everyone like him. He felt like every decision was made with the intention of gaining approval, but once he got on someone's good side, he no longer felt any attachment toward them and cut off contact. He struggled with empathy because he used to care too much and be too empathetic as a child, so he cut off his emotions as a defense mechanism. He was also so insecure and anxious that if anyone around him was more intelligent than him, it would trigger suicidal thoughts.

Now that he has developed more empathy, he begins to feel guilty about all the people he has cut off, and he is trying to be more compassionate with himself as well. He still struggles with giving sincere apologies, loving someone in a "normal" way, and accepting love from others if he feels he has not "earned" it by being the best person in the world, but he has gotten better. He reports that doing inner child work and grounding exercises are key to his recovery.

Malignant Narcissists

Malignant narcissists are the most dangerous of the bunch. They can be either overt or covert—meaning that they may be straightforward or passive-aggressive in their approach. But one fact is consistent: they are unfailingly sadistic. They put others down in order to raise themselves up and take a lot of joy in doing so. They are quick to point fingers at those who don't see them as the incredible person they believe they are, and they are likely to engage in revenge plots. Not all malignant narcissists are physically abusive, but they are more likely to use physical violence than any other type. Therapy is difficult for the malignant narcissist because they will abuse their therapist like they do everyone else, so they can be especially tricky to work with.

The concept of malignant narcissism began with Erich Fromm's theory, which closely followed Kohut's first assertions about NPD. He saw malignant narcissism as the core of many of humanity's problems, and he even went as far as to call it "the most severe pathology and the root of the most vicious destructiveness and inhumanity." Fromm believed that Adolf Hitler was a malignant narcissist, so he understood the condition as a key trait of the evilest people on earth.

Shortly after, more people began to theorize about the malignant narcissist and what it means to bear that diagnosis. Edith Weigert saw it as an escape from reality, while Herbert Rosenfeld saw it as a more aggressive form of NPD. However, Otto Kernberg noticed a bit of overlap in the symptoms of a malignant narcissist and someone with an antisocial personality disorder, so he asserted that malignant narcissism must include some element of sadism. Kernberg used the terms "malignant narcissist" and "psychopath" interchangeably in a 1970 article, which created a lot of confusion about the unique definitions of both words. In the end, we came to think of the conditions as a sliding scale, with psychopathy being the most severe, NPD as the mildest, and malignant narcissism somewhere between the two (George, 2018).

As you can see, the malignant narcissist has the worst form of NPD possible without slipping into the realm of psychopathy. Their reality is excessively warped, and they express their frustration with the world through violent means. This type of NPD is also the rarest, partially thanks to the strict requirements needed to be diagnosed as one. The following examples portray symptoms of malignant narcissism. They can be helpful when trying to understand the nature of this disorder.

Example 1: The Fight Starter

User CherryBobbins on Reddit shared the story of her narcissistic sister on December 7, 2020. The user (whom I will call Cherry) has struggled with her older sister for many years, but she says her parents have been ignoring the signs, which has been detrimental for Cherry's development. The narcissist feels entitled to everything that Cherry owns. Cherry has to protect her belongings if she does not want them to be stolen. Her sister ends multiple familial relationships if the family member does not recognize her as the perfect person that she wants to be seen as. Shortly before Cherry posted to Reddit, her sister started a fight where she called their parents "disgusting racists," and she began withholding access to her children, whom the family used to be close with.

Cherry also mentions that her sister's husband may be aware of his wife's tendencies and feels the effects of her narcissism as well. He offers the family a means of video-calling with the children without his wife knowing, but Cherry suspects that he does not have the heart to stand up to her.

Because of this narcissist's confrontational and argumentative nature, I would peg her as a malignant narcissist. She seems to have overt methods since she cuts off people who criticize her and takes pleasure in starting fights and causing her family discomfort. She may also be manipulating and abusing her husband and children.

Example 2: The Blackmail Family

This story was shared by user MathmaticianIll71711 on Reddit, though she used a throwaway account because she felt unsafe posting on her main profile. She tells us that her younger sister and mother are narcissists, and they are both violent in their own ways.

Her mother, whom she is already cut off contact with, denies the fact that she used to hit her or downplays the abuse. She says she "only hit her five times in her life," which is blatantly untrue and would still be abuse even if it "only" happened five times. Meanwhile, her narcissistic younger sister uses intimidation tactics in an attempt to keep control, threatening to tell their father that the poster is a sex worker. The poster decided to tell her father herself in order to take that power away from her narcissistic sibling.

The constant abuse from two narcissists has taken a toll on her. She reports that it takes her several days to feel normal after she is forced to interact with either of them. Moreover, she is often paranoid that she is the true narcissist.

Threats, violence, and revenge are key trademarks of a malignant narcissist, so it seems as though both family members fall into this category. They will often resort to extreme measures to maintain the hierarchy they have established, and they are careful not to give their victims any ground. They can also engage in gaslighting, which means they lead their victims to question reality or to wonder whether they are the ones who are "going crazy." This seems to have already happened to the victim, as she thinks she may be the narcissist when the evidence she has shared suggests that she is not in the wrong.

Variations in Type

As you read through those explanations and examples, you may still be having a hard time placing exactly what kind of narcissist your sibling is. They may have characteristics of multiple types, or maybe they simply don't seem to match with the examples. If that is the case, you might be wondering if there is any sort of a gray area between the three main types of narcissism.

One study suggests that some fluctuation between types may be possible, particularly between classic and vulnerable types. Some narcissists in the study who were typically classic seemed to show some tendencies toward vulnerable narcissism at different times in their life. This implies that it is possible to fluctuate somewhat between the types as time passes. Narcissists who are primarily vulnerable showed much lower rates of fluctuation, though the study admits that the concept needs to be developed further to give us a better understanding of what it means to switch between types (Edershile, 2020).

However, beyond these vague studies, there is no evidence that a person can be multiple types at once, exist somewhere between types, or combine qualities from multiple types. When theorizing about what type your sibling might be, go with whatever option seems closest to their behavior, even if the description does not match exactly. Most people are likely to be different from the textbook definitions of the types in at least a small way, so we have to go with whatever is the best fit.

Historical Narcissists

We already analyzed a large number of real-life narcissists and seen how they can affect the lives of their lovers, families, and peers. However, there is another type of example we can look at to solidify our concept of narcissism: historical narcissists. Since people with NPD (especially those of the classic type) are so likely to hold leadership positions, it is no surprise that there have been plenty of narcissists in our history books. It is absolutely astonishing to think about how our lives are so affected by narcissists, even if there is not one in our household. By simply living in a world with a social hierarchy, we are stepped on by narcissists all of the time!

However, as you continue reading, it is important to remember that most of the figures I will be talking about are not officially diagnosed. We have no solid evidence of their narcissism, but we can observe their actions, words, and personal lives to come up with a theory about whether or not they have the disorder. When placing a person on this list, I looked at a number of aspects to see where to put them. First of all, were they introverted or extroverted? If introverted, they were more likely to be vulnerable narcissists, while extroverts were probably classic. Were they manipulative, or were they physically violent? If they were violent, especially toward those who did not worship the ground they walked, I considered them malignant narcissists. Lastly, how well did they hide their narcissism? Classic narcissists are typically a little better at hiding it and may be seen by many as good businessmen or simply successful.

Historical Classic Narcissists

- **Napoleon Bonaparte:** Besides Adolf Hitler, who we discussed earlier in this book, Napoleon is the most well-known historical example of a narcissist. Napoleon believed that he was an "unusual" person who was capable of doing the impossible. In his book *Thoughts*, he wrote, "It was precisely that evening in Lodi that I came to believe in myself as an unusual person and became consumed with the ambition to do the great things that until then had been but a fantasy." He was also known for being loud, in-charge, and dominating. One of his most lasting legacies is the phrase "Napoleon complex." We use it to refer to someone who acts tough when they are actually quite small. It sounds like a clear narcissist to me!

- **Ronald Reagan:** Jeffrey Kluger, the author of *The Narcissist Next Door*, calls Reagan "perhaps the most highly functional narcissist who's ever been in [the American] political system." Whatever you think about him and his politics, you have to admit that he had an abundance of confidence and seemed comfortable in everything he did. Since he was always so high-functioning, it is easy to place him in the classic category. History has portrayed him in a lot of different ways. Some see him as the best president in our recent history, while others say that he was a complete menace. Either way, Reagan's opinion of himself would likely go unchanged (Kluger, 2019).

- **Madonna:** Before anyone gets upset upon seeing her name on his list, you might be interested to hear that Madonna has called herself a narcissist. She actually cites it as a major factor behind her success. If she didn't love being in the center of the room and being exhibitionistic, do you think she would be as big of a figure as she is? Since she is extremely successful in her career and also very upfront about her personality, it only makes sense to think of her as a classic narcissist (Davies, 2017).

Historical Vulnerable Narcissists

- **Bill Clinton:** Like all vulnerable narcissists, Clinton has a self-destructive nature hidden behind a wall of charisma, charm, and generosity. Unfortunately for him, the whole country's eyes were on him, and his downfall was extremely public. And despite all of that, many people in the American population still forgave him, presumably because of his immense charm and docile nature. Although we don't get a close look into the daily lives of the American presidents, I would love to see just how all of the negative publicity affected him as a vulnerable narcissist (Kluger, 2019).

- **Henry VIII:** This infamous monarch is a little hard to classify into a type, especially because of his personality shift after his concussion, but I am placing him on the vulnerable list because of his inherent paranoia and his anger when criticized. Henry VIII, best known for his six wives, also executed 57,000 people during his reign, mostly in fits of anger. He was also obsessed over his looks, which may have started with his sudden weight gain in his adulthood after spending his youth as a handsome, lean young man. He also created an entire church so that he could get his way, which is a feat only a narcissist could pull (Lessons From History, 2020).

Historical Malignant Narcissists

- **Alexander the Great:** No one should be surprised to see Alexander on this list. This man saw himself as the "new Achilles" and obsessed over recreating the myth's image in reality. He opted for the Persian style of kingship, rather than the Macedonian style his father enjoyed, because it was more lavish and made him feel he was being worshipped. Speaking of his father, his false self was so overpowering that he convinced himself that his true father was Zeus, not King Phillip II of Macedonia. He conquered many, many lands in his own name and with lots of bloodsheds, including that of his closest friends. If he suspected them of being traitors or if they criticized him in any way, he had them killed (Lessons From History,

2020). His methods were very assertive and confident, so I am willing to peg him as an overt malignant narcissist.

- **Nero:** Most people know about Nero's persecution of Christians, which is why Nero is on the malignant end of the spectrum, but they may not know about his attempts at godhood. He killed his mother when she showed interest in taking some of his power, and he constantly bad-mouthed the rest of his family. He was also, to be frank, obnoxious. He believed he was a great musician despite having no real skill, so he forced others to listen to his performances for hours and hours. He also participated in the Olympics, which he always won because no one can tell their emperor "no," and hosted a festival called Neronia that only existed so that he could win prizes in poetry and music. However, the people saw past him, and the army revolted, so apparently, the image he constructed was not nearly solid enough (Lessons From History, 2020). Since he mostly used manipulative means and lies to convince others of his greatness, I believe he may be a covert malignant narcissist.

Somatic vs. Cerebral

So far, we have been talking a lot about the three main types and how they relate to being covert or overt. We know that classic narcissists must be overt, vulnerable narcissists must be covert, and malignant narcissists could be either. However, there is another classification that can be applied to all three main types of NPD: somatic vs. cerebral narcissism.

As we have already discussed, a somatic narcissist is someone who values their looks, while a cerebral narcissist is someone who values their mind. It seems fairly clear-cut, but there can actually be a lot of variance in these two subtypes.

Sam Vaknin is a cerebral narcissist who explains the key differences and similarities of these subtypes in his article "Dr. Jackal and Mr. Hide (Somatic vs. Cerebral Narcissists)." As he puts it, all narcissists have both somatic and cerebral traits inside of them but are likely to have a preference toward one or the other. He also believes that it is possible to switch between being somatic and cerebral at different stages of a narcissist's life, which he claims to have done. Although he considers himself a cerebral narcissist most of the time, his somatic side has risen to the surface during and after the most difficult stages of his life, as though it was being used as a coping mechanism. He also states that both types are autoerotic—meaning that they are in love with their own bodies and minds and that the dominant type can be determined by their approach to sex (Vaknin, 2018). Let us see what he has to say about what a narcissist's libido ultimately reveals about them.

Somatic Narcissists

As Vaknin describes, the somatic narcissist is often a very sexual person. They may enjoy flaunting their bodies, which they take great care into maintaining, to any partners who are willing to see it and take a great deal of pride in their sexual performance. However, behind the showmanship, the somatic narcissist is actually quite emotionally distant from the act of sex and is unlikely to form much of a bond with their partners. They see the act of physical intimacy as a form of masturbation, where their partner is simply a toy they use to satisfy their own desires and stroke their own egos. Our sex-crazed culture often normalizes this mindset, especially through our music and video games, so many people around the narcissist may not even notice the problem or think it is unusual at all, but even the narcissist themselves might feel that something is off. Since they approach sex with a self-serving, superficial sort of mindset, they might find that sex becomes unfulfilling. It may feel empty and even draining, but they may keep trying in the hopes that next time will be "different."

Furthermore, a somatic narcissist is probably very vocal about their sex lives and will take any opportunity they can to talk about it, even if it feels inappropriate. When you think about this subtype, it may help to imagine some of our favorite celebrities, such as Kanye West, Kim Kardashian, and more. They are flashy, larger-than-life trendsetters, but something about their behavior feels a little detached. They don't really care about the people they pursue, even if it feels romantic. It is all about themselves and their fame (Vaknin, 2018).

Cerebral Narcissists

On the opposite side of the spectrum is the cerebral narcissist. This subtype is unlikely to care about sex at all. In fact, they may be sex-repulsed or voluntarily celibate. Sometimes they simply don't think about sex and romance because they are too engaged in their intellectual endeavors. They use their mind as a means of securing adoration and praise, regardless of how intelligent they really are. Even if they are simply average or below average, they will go to great lengths to make you believe otherwise. They will cheat to achieve different accomplishments and awards, thrive on praises, and bring their successes up in any way they can.

This does not mean that the cerebral narcissist has no libido at all—they are just more likely to turn to pornography and masturbation as a means of quickly squelching their cravings instead of seeking a partner. Masturbation may feel like a bit of a chore to them, a necessary evil to help them focus on whatever they have set their minds to.

If they lack any somatic traits, maintenance of their body may be seen as a burden to them, and they may be annoyed by the constant need to make meals, exercise, and groom to take care of their bodies. However, it is also very possible for the cerebral narcissist to continue caring a great deal about their bodies and believe that their bodies are aesthetically pleasing to look at, even if they don't have sex extremely often. They may take some pride in being beautiful but untouchable, or they might look down on others who have sex more frequently and use it as a sign of their intellectual superiority (Vaknin, 2018).

Fluctuations

As I was reading through Vaknin's descriptions of these two subtypes, I found myself more and more interested in his personal experience with narcissism and how he found himself fluctuating between dominantly somatic and dominantly cerebral traits. As he describes, he had a number of life crises: a divorce, prison time, fleeing countries as a refugee, and large monetary losses. He was harassed, stalked, threatened, and insulted on many different occasions.

After each of these life-changing events, he switched from a cerebral to a somatic narcissist. In his own words:

> I became a lascivious lecher. When this happened, I had a few relationships—

replete with abundant and addictive
sex—going simultaneously. I
participated in and initiated group sex
and mass orgies. I exercised, lost weight,
and honed my body into an irresistible
proposition. This outburst of
unrestrained, primordial lust waned in a
few months, and I settled back into my
cerebral ways. No sex, no women, no
body. (Vaknin, 2018)

After he switched back to his usual cerebral behaviors,
his partners at the time found themselves stunned at
the change. From their point of view, their sexual
companion suddenly abandoned his body and all
pursuits of pleasure. Did they think he was depressed?
Did they think he lost interest in them? Did they take it
personally?

Regardless of the partners' interpretation of Vaknin's
actions, Vaknin himself sees this as a natural fluctuation
that takes place in the lives of most narcissists. Take a
moment to consider your sibling's life, particularly their
past relationships. Have they ever appeared to lose
interest in their partner very quickly? Have they ever
started a diet, only to abandon it shortly after and not
seem to care about their bodies as much? On the flip
side, is your sibling someone who is very interested in
their appearance but goes through phases of forgetting
basic hygiene? These fluctuations may not only point to
them being narcissists but also indicate that they are
going through a major life shift and have temporarily

fluctuated to their secondary subtype as they cope with it (Vaknin, 2018).

Chapter 4:
What Makes a Narcissist?

Everyone falls for the villain. As we watch our favorite television shows and movies, we are always waiting to hear about the motive of the villain and are hoping to be absolutely spellbound by their story. Do they have a tragic backstory or a radical philosophy that makes too much sense to be comfortable? Do they simply thrive in the chaos, or are they some personification of evil? Whatever their reason is, our media has taught us that everyone has reasons behind their actions, even if it is not a part of the main storyline.

People with NPD are not villains; they are people. It is important to keep their humanity and emotions in mind as you learn to live with them, but we can also keep that lesson in mind as we contemplate what makes a narcissist.

Chapter 1 briefly discussed three main reasons why someone might develop NPD and how these factors combine via the diathesis stress model. This chapter will go into more detail about all these ideas and look at some first-hand analyses from diagnosed narcissists about why they believe they developed the disorder.

Genetics vs. Environment

There is strong evidence to suggest that NPD and the other 10 personality disorders are at least moderately hereditary. If a person is born to a narcissistic parent, they are more likely to become a narcissist themselves. Naturally, you may already be seeing some difficulties in quantifying this; if a person was raised by a narcissist, they might have been abused themselves, right? This slips back into the territory of environmental factors, doesn't it?

Well, it is complicated. Before we look at some studies, let me explain some context behind the three clusters of personality disorder.

The Three Clusters: A, B, and C

We can look at each of the symptoms of the 10 personality disorders identified in the DSM-5 and split them into three different categories. These clusters all share some similar traits and are sometimes confused for one another, so having these clusters helps a psychiatrist to recognize the similarities and give the most accurate diagnosis. The clusters are as follows:

Cluster A: Eccentric Personality Disorders

- Schizoid personality disorder
- Schizotypal personality disorder
- Paranoid personality disorder

Cluster A personality disorders all share a quality of oddness. They are frequently outcast by society and seen as bizarre. Depending on the severity of the disorder, strangers may notice their symptoms and think something is off about them. For example, schizotypal individuals sometimes hear voices, believe that everyday things have "messages" for them, and believe that their thoughts have magical qualities. They are also likely to dress, speak, and act in unusual ways.

Cluster B: Dramatic Personality Disorders

- Borderline personality disorder
- Antisocial personality disorder
- Histrionic personality disorder
- Narcissistic personality disorder

Cluster B personality disorders are the group we will be looking at most often as it contains NPD. Along with the other disorders in the cluster, NPD has very dramatic, unpredictable, and often exaggerated symptoms. They all struggle to maintain relationships because of this, as we know from our studies of NPD. The other disorders in this cluster are similar. For example, people with histrionic personality disorder have sudden, violent outbursts as a means of gaining attention.

Cluster C: Anxious Personality Disorders

- Obsessive-compulsive personality disorder
- Dependent personality disorder
- Avoidant personality disorder

People who have one of the cluster C personality disorders have an underlying fear that has created their disorder. They will often go to great lengths to avoid this fear and require a lot of recovery time after being exposed to it. For instance, people with a dependent personality disorder fear being alone and having to take care of themselves, so they will often remain in unhealthy relationships just to avoid being alone. Meanwhile, people with avoidant personality disorder fear rejection and failure. They avoid human contact in general so that disappointing them remains an impossibility (Behavioral Health Florida, 2020).

Genetic Disposition Between Clusters

One study led by Tom Reichborn-Kjennerud, Ph.D., shows that all 10 personality disorders are at least moderately genetic. Also, their comorbidity rates are not restricted to the cluster they are assigned to in the DSM-5.

Those comorbidity rates are extremely high. If a person is diagnosed with one personality disorder, they most likely have another. The common belief is that people tend to have disorders only within a single cluster and inherit disorders from that same cluster, but that is not always the case. In fact, there seems to be a very strong connection between paranoid personality disorder, histrionic personality disorder, borderline personality disorder, dependent personality disorder, obsessive-compulsive personality disorder, and narcissistic personality disorder. People with NPD have a high chance of also developing one of those other disorders, and they are capable of inheriting NPD from a family member who has any of those personality disorders. In general, people have a 24 percent chance of inheriting narcissism, and the study found no significant correlation between sex, environmental differences, or any other outside factor (Torgerson, 2012).

What this study tells us is that if there is a narcissist in your family, there is a chance that someone else in the previous generation has a personality disorder as well. Their disorder does not necessarily have to be NPD; the simple existence of another person with a personality disorder (most likely paranoid, histrionic, borderline, or dependent) increases a person's chances of developing narcissism. Likewise, someone with NPD is more likely to have a comorbidity with one of those four other disorders. Although we have previously thought of comorbidities as conditions that are in the same cluster, those personality disorders are scattered among all of the three clusters, so the separation bears no difference when determining genetics and comorbidities.

More Statistics and Comorbidities

Since narcissism and other personality disorders have a high rate of being inherited, there must be populations that are more affected by it than others, right? That is exactly what a study by the Journal of Clinical Psychiatry was determined to discover. This study consisted of face-to-face interviews with 34,653 adults, and it gave us some very interesting statistics about the kinds of people who have NPD.

Although Reichborn-Kjennerud's study found no significant difference between the genders of people with NPD when it comes to inheritance and comorbidity, this study suggests that males are, on average, more likely to develop the disorder—4.8 percent of women in the study had NPD while 7.7 percent of men had it. According to Stinson (2008), of these people, these are the populations that have a higher prevalence of the disorder than average:

- Black men and women
- Hispanic women
- Young adults
- Separated/divorced/widowed/single adults
- Men with mental disability

- People with substance abuse problems, mood disorders, other personality disorders, and anxiety
- Women with specific phobias, anxiety, and bipolar II disorder
- Men who struggle with alcohol abuse and dependency
- People without dysthymia

That last population is fairly interesting. Dysthymia is a mild but often long-lasting form of depression that includes symptoms of low mood, low energy, low sleep, low appetite, poor concentration, and loss of interest in normal activities. It is sometimes called persistent depressive disorder because of its long-lasting nature; the diagnosis requires at least two years of symptoms (Mayo Clinic, 2018).

The study shows that people with NPD were significantly less likely to suffer from dysthymia than other populations, and the reason for this is unknown. The authors suggest one theory about the men in the study: since men also had high rates of substance abuse, it is possible that men with NPD tend to self-medicate with drugs and alcohol to fight the symptoms associated with dysthymia. However, this theory does not explain why women with NPD do not experience dysthymia, so more research may be needed to discern why this correlation exists (Stinson, 2008).

Twin Studies

When we covered the diathesis stress model in chapter 1, we learned that most individuals with a genetic predisposition toward NPD still need to have the trait triggered in some way in order to start displaying symptoms. It is extremely difficult to measure the impact of genetics versus environment when all people have different genes since the variables are too unpredictable. However, there is one instance where people can have the same genes with potentially different upbringings—twins.

Twin studies involve examining twins who have been separated at birth or have been raised in different environments for any variety of reasons. Since they have the same genes, we have the freedom to examine their environments alone.

One twin study led by Yu L Luo, Huajian Cai, and Hairong Song in 2014 looked into 304 pairs of twins in Beijing to examine the main traits associated with narcissism—intrapersonal grandiosity and interpersonal entitlement. The life circumstances of these twins were primarily unique: 92–93 percent of the twins had different living environments from their siblings. This study is unique as it allows us to look at the heritability of the different aspects of narcissism rather than the disorder at large. The results are extremely interesting: intrapersonal grandiosity has a 23 percent chance of being inherited, while interpersonal entitlement has a 35 percent chance of being inherited. It shows that these aspects can express themselves independently in an individual with a genetic predisposition (Luo, 2014).

A different twin study in 2006 led by the American Journal of Psychiatry examined 175 twin pairs and questioned them on the criteria for narcissism with the intention of seeing how narcissism compares with other personality traits. Submissiveness and attachment problems had very low heritability, but narcissistic characteristics had up to 64% heritability. As the study reports, that number is similar to the heritability to normal personality traits, suggesting that NPD is as inheritable as personality traits outside of the disorder, such as introversion, extroversion, and more (American Journal of Psychiatry, 2006).

These twin studies have illustrated a few different notable factors that make a narcissist. They both prove the potent heritability of the disorder as well as the individual symptoms that define it. They also show that the environment plays a large part in ultimately determining if a person will have NPD. As suggested in chapter 1, these two elements work together to create a narcissist.

Technology and Narcissism

When we think about our environment and how we were raised, we typically imagine how our parents treated us, how we were viewed by our extended family, and how we managed our early lives in school. It is undeniable that these elements play a large part in how our minds change and grow, but the modern world has thrown in a new complication to our social lives: technology.

With the rise of social media, young people are now able to communicate with people all across the world. They can share selfies, status updates, and opinions, and they can even chat with people they will never see in person. I am not here to talk badly about technology; our advancements have done a lot of good for our world and changed a lot of lives for the better. However, is it completely unreasonable to hypothesize that technology has changed the way that conditions like narcissism are triggered?

According to a study held by Intentions Consulting, a market research firm, that hypothesis hits the nail on the head. This study surveyed 2,025 Americans and asked them a series of questions about their mental health, stressors, and diagnosed disorders while also gaining information about how much screen time they have each day. The findings were telling; young people who spend more time on social media are more stressed about finances, family, and work. They feel more isolated from others, believe that people are judging them, and even worry more about others trying to hurt them. It also found out that spending more than four hours a day on social media, apps, and other online platforms makes a person 31 percent more likely to develop NPD.

Four hours sounds like a long time, but in reality, most Americans between ages 16 and 24 spend more than double that time on social media: a whopping 8.5 hours (Badminton, 2020). Suddenly, the statistics from earlier stating that young adults have a higher rate of NPD makes a lot more sense.

But technology is meant to bring us closer together, right? How is social media supposed to make us even more antisocial? Well, the problem with social media is that it creates a very me-centric environment. YouTube and TikTok only recommend videos that the algorithm believes you will like. Twitter and Facebook only expose you to friends of friends and allow you to block anyone you don't like. Even the advertisements you receive on a variety of platforms are catered to your specific interests. Social media gives the illusion of making you more cultured, but it actually keeps you limited to a small corner of the World Wide Web (Elgan, 2009).

Jean Twenge was the lead author of a study that shows college students have been getting more and more narcissistic since 1982. This study dealt with a questionnaire that asked students whether they agreed with statements such as "The world would be a better place if I ruled it," "I am above average in everything that I do," and more. When this study was completed in 2007, about two-thirds of students scored above average, implying that they are more self-centered and less empathetic.

Twenge suggests that this rise of narcissism began with the "self-esteem movement" of the '80s, where children were encouraged to think highly of themselves in the hopes of battling depression (NPR, 2007). I believe that Twenge may be onto something. That movement likely affected many people when they were young, especially those who were raised in the '80s, but our teens have been subjected to so much more since that time. In fact, social media has become more centric in our lives since 2007, the time of that study. I believe that technology has a major role in the results of that questionnaire and will only cause more damage as time progresses.

As you try to understand your sibling, consider the ways that technology has influenced your lives and how your sibling uses technology. Do they spend most of their day browsing content specific to their interests? Do they post a lot of selfies, statuses, and milestones on Facebook? Do they lack hobbies outside of watching YouTube, using TikTok, and playing video games? Has this behavior been a pattern since they were young? Have they ever been cyberbullied, or do they cyberbully others? With the rise of technology, it is important to consider our digital environment as well as our physical one.

Brain Structure

Although genetics and environment tend to take the forefront of the discussion, there is another important factor that can potentially make a narcissist: brain structure. Recently, psychologists have been looking at how the actual makeup of the brain affects different disorders, and NPD is no exception. Through different studies and MRI scans, we have learned a lot about how a narcissist's brain differs from that of a healthy individual.

A team of scientists led by Dr. Stefan Röpke in 2013 analyzed a group of 34 people, 17 of whom were diagnosed narcissists. By comparing the people with NPD to those without it, the scientists were able to notice a major difference: the thickness of the cerebral cortex. The cerebral cortex is a thin layer of the brain that covers the cerebrum, and it is sometimes called the gray matter because its lack of insulation gives it a gray shade. The cerebral cortex is important for a number of functions, including personality, intelligence, motor function, ability to plan, language processing, and more. Damages to the cerebral cortex can result in Alzheimer's, Parkinson's, and even depression. The cerebral cortex also controls an ability that narcissists struggle with: compassion (Bailey, 2020).

Interestingly, the participants who had NPD had a notably thinner cerebral cortex in comparison to the control group. Here's what Dr. Röpke, head of the study, had to say about the results:

> Our data shows that the amount of empathy is directly correlated to the volume of gray brain matter of the corresponding cortical representation in the insular region, and that the patients with narcissism exhibit a structural deficit in exactly this area. Building on this initial structural data, we are currently attempting to use functional imaging (fMRI) to understand better how the brains of patients with narcissistic personality disorder work.

Another study from 2010 looked at brain activity rather than brain structure. The volunteer test subjects were instructed to complete a series of activities while their brain was monitored, and they were also observed during the rest period between activities. Most of these test subjects were healthy and did not have an NPD diagnosis, but like all of us, they had varying degrees of narcissistic traits.

Their findings were unique. Those who had higher levels of narcissistic traits, such as pridefulness and arrogance, had more brain activity during rest periods. The activity was occurring specifically in a part of the cerebral cortex responsible for self-absorbed thinking, as well as an area associated with impulsive decisions. This tells us that people who are more self-obsessed, such as a narcissist, are more likely to make poor decisions (Ranch TN, 2013).

A final study looked not at the brain itself but at the blood that cycles through the brain. This study was hosted by Dr. Royce Lee, a psychiatrist and personality disorder specialist at the University of Chicago Medicine. It took a look at the oxidative stress in the blood of people with narcissistic personality disorder.

Oxidative stress is defined as a molecular imbalance between antioxidants and free radicals in the body. This imbalance puts a lot of stress on the body because it requires the body to metabolize the excess oxidative chemicals as it cycles through the brain and the rest of the limbs. The study found an excess of the molecule 8-OH-DG, a biomarker of oxidative stress. These results were extremely similar to those found in individuals with borderline personality disorder (BPD). This is especially interesting since BPD is associated with chronically low self-esteem, the exact opposite of NPD. However, despite their differences, it seems as though the two conditions are biologically similar.

The study also emphasizes that although narcissists may appear cold and uncaring, they are actually hypersensitive to their surroundings. As Lee, the head of the study, puts it:

> We found that the levels of oxidative stress were related to impaired recognition or expression of shame. That is interesting because we know

from previous research that people high
in narcissism have problems with the
emotion of shame. What we are trying
to figure out is the relationship between
hypersensitivity and shame and why that
leads people to avoid empathy. This
paper does not quite get us there. That
is the next question.

As Lee made clear in his statement, there are still a lot
of questions about the biological factors involved in
NPD and the other nine personality disorders. We are
constantly making discoveries, and these steps forward
help to give us hope that people who are burdened by
NPD will be able to receive better treatment in the
future.

Real-Life Examples

If your sibling's narcissism has gone untreated for a
long time and has absorbed their true selves, they are
unlikely to talk to you (or anyone else) about how they
developed their narcissism. In fact, they probably don't
even recognize that they have a problem and will
become defensive or aggressive if you try to bring it up.
It often takes a lot of treatment to help a narcissist
understand how flawed their view of reality is, so you
probably will not hear your sibling's story from their
own mouths in quite some time. And if you do, you
can't trust that it has not been confabulated or

exaggerated to fill in the memory gaps of their dissociation.

Thankfully, we can hear the stories of different narcissists who have been undergoing therapy and have a clearer idea of how their disorder took root. The following stories were shared by diagnosed narcissists on Reddit who have a suspicion of where their lives took a turn for the worse. As you read them, think about what you know of your sibling and what may have caused their warped perception to set in.

Example 1: Emotional Loneliness

Reddit user Literallytwodaysold reports having a bit of genetic predisposition to the condition, but we know that genetics alone is not always enough to create a narcissist. She cites emotional loneliness as the primary cause, alongside her genetics.

Although all her physical needs were fulfilled beyond what she could ever ask for, she was left alone when it came to emotional needs. Her family never talked about feelings, so she navigated her emotions on her own and ended up developing a narcissistic "reward system" without realizing that her mindset was toxic. Since no one talked to her about emotions, she didn't know that what she was doing was abnormal, and having a high number of narcissists in her family gave her a skewed vision of how most people handle themselves.

Her story goes to show how a family has responsibilities to their children beyond just their physical needs, especially when the child is already at-risk for NPD because of her genetics.

Example 2: Love and Abuse

Reddit user Ambrose_1987Sep30, a covert narcissist, shares his story about how a combination of suffocating love and overwhelming abuse caused his NPD. He does not believe there are any other narcissists in his family, so he looked to environmental factors to help determine the cause of his disorder.

When he was in preschool, he was treated exceptionally well by his parents but was molested by his uncle. As he entered elementary school, his parents began to suspect that he would grow up to be gay. They started vocally expressing their disgust toward gay people, insulting flamboyant characters on television, and making overall closed-minded statements as an attempt to discourage the tendencies they saw in him. However, their words did not change his sexuality. They made him realize that their love was conditional and that he would not be accepted if he ever came out. It also caused him to obsess over being perfect, which planted those narcissistic thoughts in his mind.

He states that his parents' overwhelming love, their hatred toward his sexuality, and the abuse from his uncle were the main contributing factors to his NPD.

He wonders if he would be a different type of narcissist or if he would have ever developed NPD in the first place if not for one of those elements.

Example 3: Neglect and Insecurity

Gothonaut on Reddit posted in December 2020 that her narcissism was caused by a combination of neglect from both parents, insecurity in familial and platonic relationships, and only being recognized for her looks.

Her family divorced when she was only four years old, and her father was absent from then forward. Her mom was emotionally closed off and often away at her job, where she worked long shifts as a nurse. She was an only child, and most of her friendships were extremely rocky, so she would have no company for most of her days. In fact, the only attention she received was in response to her looks since she was a beautiful child.

In response, she became an attention-seeker with an innate inability to trust. Childhood neglect is a common theme among narcissists, and she also fell into this trap as she attempted to raise herself. With nothing but media and the internet to create her morals, it is no surprise that she fell into a toxic mindset and is still in recovery. I am interested to hear her relationship with technology, especially as someone who was highly recognized for her appearance. Influencers on Instagram are given special treatment for just being pretty, so maybe her young mind assumed that she should be the same.

Example 4: Familial Lineage

This story comes from Butterfun02 on Reddit. The poster herself is not a narcissist, but her mother was, and she came to learn a lot about her mother's traumatic past.

The narcissistic mother's dad was a World War II veteran who became an abusive alcoholic. He was controlling over his wife, forbidding her from talking to other men or even getting coffee with some other women at church. In one of the scarier stories the Redditor heard about him, he came home drunk one evening, accused his wife of having an affair, and stormed around the house, firing a shotgun at random. In the meantime, their two children hid underneath a bed to protect themselves. Both of those children, an older sister and a younger brother, would grow up to be narcissists.

The older sister ended up being very socially distant from the rest of her family. Although the younger brother was more beloved by their parents, he inherited his father's alcoholism and struggled with it for most of his life. The older sister also may have had a minor cognitive disorder, as reported by her daughter. This falls in line with some of the statistics we already looked at. Narcissists are more likely to have mental disability or substance abuse problems, particularly men.

The Redditor also tells us that she did better in school than her mother, which might have spawned a lot of jealousy and become a potential motive behind some abuse. As a narcissist, she probably struggled to have a daughter who was more intellectually accomplished than her.

The narcissist's daughter also shares some closing thoughts with us:

> Sometimes appearances can be deceiving about their upbringings. My mom always talked about what great parents she had. But then she would describe the things they did. Or after she died, I heard about the beatings. But she called them "good Christian people." I feel like trauma and neglect are at play in most [narcissists] I know.

Although we don't know the grandfather's full story, I believe he may have some sort of personality disorder outside of any post-traumatic stress he may have gained during the war. His controlling, violent nature is not normal, and there may be some level of manipulation involved since his daughter still considered him a good parent. If he did have a personality disorder, perhaps it contributed a bit of genetic risk to his children as well. His son inherited his alcoholism, so maybe he also inherited a personality disorder. Either way, the abuse those two children endured and witnessed was horrendous and would have a strong impact on anyone who lived through something like that. Trauma and neglect is certainly a common theme in the stories we have examined.

Chapter 5:

Living With Narcissists

It is so easy to feel alone when you are dealing with a narcissist. Not only are you dealing with constant manipulation and aggression, but the gaslighting makes you believe that you are simply being dramatic or that you are the true narcissist. When you talk to others about what you are experiencing, they tell you that it is simply how siblings treat each other. However, you know that something is inherently wrong with what you are going through. There is some sort of deeper issue at play here, even if you are the only one who is willing to recognize it.

Hopefully, reading through the real-life examples in the last few chapters helped you to understand that you are not actually alone. There are more narcissists in our world than we think, and there are even more now than there were 40 years ago. Each of these narcissists has a family, and many of them have siblings that they have abused for years and years.

However, sharing real-life stories of narcissists has a major downfall that I have already addressed a few times: I can't be sure of their exact diagnosis, the ins and outs of their behavior, and the full context of the situations described over the internet. To remedy this major inadequacy, I would like to spend a chapter constructing realistic but imaginary narcissists and their families. I will use major patterns in narcissistic behavior, the requirements for the diagnosis, and my own personal experience with narcissists to fabricate each scenario and give you a full breakdown of each character. This way, you will have a complete idea of how a narcissist might think.

Some of these stories might look like an exact portrait of your sibling, but it is equally possible that none of them will. No worries; all people are different, and everyone who shares a diagnosis does not express their symptoms in the same way. However, knowing how to give a complete analysis of a handful of fictional narcissists will certainly help you to have a full understanding of the seemingly mysterious actions of NPD.

Classic Narcissist

Imagine a typical country home in Maine. The suburbs are beautiful, especially in the autumn and winter, and the town is a popular tourist destination for those who like to hike, fish, or are simply craving a little bit more nature in their lives.

Peter, however, seems to see no real beauty outside of himself. He just turned 17 in the summer, and his birthday party was elaborate and enormous. He invited all of the soccer team, their girlfriends, and a few other buddies from class who did not seem to fit in as well, but they were extremely grateful to have been invited regardless. All in all, there were about 20 people there, bopping around to play soccer in the backyard, enjoy some fruit punch, and give Peter his gifts.

There was also Peter's little brother, Evan, who kept to the sidelines. He was only 13 and didn't know too many of the older kids, so he resigned himself to an afternoon on the patio, where he could sit quickly. Frankly, a lot of the soccer boys intimidated him, especially since Evan was a bit of a late bloomer and looked like he was leagues younger than everyone there. It was uncomfortable for him, but he had confidence that he could deal with it for at least a single day.

On the plus side, at least he did not have to interact with Peter much since all of his friends were around. The two of them never got along extremely well, which Evan found disappointing. They could have been quite the dynamic duo: Peter is the brawn, Evan is the brain, and all of Maine is their playground. However, Peter seems to insist that he is both brain and brawn. About a year back, Peter convinced their parents that Evan cheated on his finals and that he would not have gotten his impressive 3.9 GPA if he had not written the answers on his wrists, which led to a long grounding and the loss of his reputation as a gifted kid. Now, everyone sees Peter as the golden child and Evan as some sort of delinquent. As he sat there at the party, he prayed that no one remembered what happened a year ago. The best-case scenario was that he would go unnoticed for the whole day while also fulfilling his obligation to attend his brother's party.

However, he had no such luck. Within 30 minutes or so, a few of the older kids noticed the tiny 13-year-old sitting alone and thought it would be polite to go talk to him. He was hesitant to tell them that he is Peter's little brother out of fear that they would remember the "cheating" incident, but they must've been new friends of Peter's because they didn't bring anything up. Evan has a hard time keeping track of Peter's friends since he cycles through them so quickly, so at least he was safe with this small group that approached them. It was a squad of three: a soccer player, his girlfriend, and her best friend.

They made courteous small talk for a while. They seemed interested in Evan's extracurricular activities and wondered if he was going to join a sport's team like his brother, but Evan told them that he was more interested in the student government. As soon as the words left his mouth, they seemed so excited for him. The soccer player was already plotting his election strategy, the girls were talking about making posters, and all of them wanted to know what he would do about the school lunches. Their excitement caused a bit of a ruckus, and they ended up attracting a small crowd of interested teenagers, none of which seemed to remember anything about Evan from last year. For a small moment, Evan could convince himself to show a little confidence and assert his opinions about the hall pass, and he was glad to hear that the other kids agreed with him.

He should have known better than to think his moment in the spotlight could last for very long. Peter must've noticed that his little brother was getting a lot of attention and burst in to ruin it. He had his best smile, his most effective charms, and all the best words, and he used them to destroy any semblance of normalcy that Evan might have had. Within minutes, he told everyone that Evan was a cheater and manipulator, that they would be safer to leave him alone, and that he had no future in student government or in any other extracurricular. However, he managed to say so in a way that made him look like a concerned friend and not a jealous older brother.

A few months passed after the birthday party, and Peter still seemed to harbor some negative feelings toward his little brother. They did not share too many peaceful, brotherly moments before, but they have become rarer and rarer. Their interactions are brief and cold.

Here's the worst part, though: Peter ran for a position on the student government. He applied the first day that it opened, and now, if Evan applied as well, he would look like the copycat. Evan is heartbroken, and when he tries to talk to his father about the problem, he dismisses it and says he was "just like Peter when he was his age."

Analysis

Peter will be familiar to many readers of this book. He is a classic narcissist to a tee—extroverted, assertive, quick to brag, and in constant need of the spotlight. He can't even stand to see his brother having attention for a few minutes as he talked to Peter's friends. The incident sparked a revenge plot that involved stealing his goals so that they would be ruined and Evan would not get more attention through a position on the student council.

It seems that Peter is actually very threatened by Evan's success. Although Peter is more skilled when it comes to social interactions and physical prowess, the cerebral narcissist in him makes him want to be seen as the more intelligent sibling as well. Since he can't compete with Evan's brain, he is forced to sabotage his little brother by lying about Evan being a cheater and by ruining Evan's goals. He will do his best to suppress those talents from showing so that he will appear to be the smarter brother. Like many people with NPD, his sense of self-worth comes from comparing himself with others, and Evan has become the primary person to draw comparisons with.

It is also very clear that Peter's main mode of expression is overt. He didn't hesitate to stand up in front of a crowd and ruin Evan's reputation, which a vulnerable narcissist might struggle to do. His confidence and straightforward nature make him an overt narcissist. This can also be seen in his false self.

The image he projects of himself is kind, fun, intelligent, and protective of his friends. He has everyone convinced that he is trying to save them from his manipulative brother, painting Evan as a vulnerable narcissist, although he is not.

The father's comment about being similar to Peter may lead us to believe that there are some hereditary factors at play here. Even if the father himself does not have NPD, he may have several narcissistic traits or perhaps a different personality disorder that leads him to relate to his eldest son. It seems that Peter has had a fairly stable childhood, but he may have felt threatened by Evan's intelligence from early on and developed low self-esteem. He then used narcissism to cope with it. It also seems that Peter has had tumultuous friendships, which could have led him to have a skewed understanding of what it means to be a friend or perhaps given him an innate distrust of others. Also, although their father seems to favor Peter, he may be distant when Peter shows any signs of weakness, just like he is with Evan, which taught him that he needs to be perfect (or at least perceived as perfect) to be worthy of his father's pride.

Vulnerable Narcissist

Marie and her little sister Anne have lived in France their whole lives, and in their youth, they used to enjoy frequent trips to Germany, Italy, England, and more.

They were both very introverted girls and tended to stick by their mother's side the whole trip. However, they still loved to see the different sights, learn about history at all the different museums, and explore the cultures in other countries. They were both very intelligent, partly thanks to their frequent travel and partly because of their mother's constant devotion. She taught them to prioritize school, encouraged them to think about their careers as a passion, and showed utmost faith in both of her daughter's abilities.

Unfortunately, everything went upside down in 2002. Marie was nine, and Anne was seven at the time, so they did not have the best understanding of what it meant for their parents to have a divorce. However, they knew that it was going to change their lives for the worse. Their mother, who was once a stay-at-home mom, was forced to find a job on her own and ended up working at a grocery store for a fairly low wage. The trips stopped, the museums became too expensive, and the overall quality of the girls' lives decreased a drastic amount.

Their mom refused to give the details of why their father left, but Marie had her suspicions. She heard them fighting after bedtime. They did their best to keep quiet and sometimes moved the conversation outside before it turned to screaming, but Marie could still hear them through the window. It sounded like her father would have sudden fits of anger where he would accuse his wife of cheating, stealing his money, or talking badly of him to her family and children. This was very upsetting for Marie because she knew her mother would not do any of these things, so she did not understand where these thoughts came from.

However, regardless of whether or not her mom did anything wrong, their father was soon out of the picture. The girls continued trying to prioritize school. They had to transfer to a cheaper institution, and Anne struggled to adjust. She was bullied at the new school and had few friends, and her mood seemed to drop. It was a miracle that she could keep her grades up despite all of this.

Anne also started to act out. If Marie was successful in school, Anne would talk about how she "might as well die because mom likes her better anyway." When Marie got a boyfriend, Anne felt that she was unlovable and was bitter about the new relationship. With every success, Anne found some way to make Marie feel guilty about it, as though she was leaving her little sister behind.

It was confusing, too, because Anne was still a very sweet girl. In fact, she sometimes gave too much of herself and was frequently burnt out, but no amount of convincing could get her to stop giving. She was quick to cut off new friends when she was able to make them, as though she was sentencing herself to a life of loneliness. It was hard for Marie to try to do anything for herself because she felt like she was taking advantage of a sad, lonely, and kind little girl who had a lot of things taken from her. Marie started to wonder if she was the narcissist after all.

Analysis

Anne is a clear-cut vulnerable narcissist, and she is especially good at manipulation. Like many others in this type, she has convinced that other people are the ones in the wrong and that she is the helpless victim. She is unable to feel empathy like a healthy individual, and it shows in the way that she can't be happy for Marie's successes. She attempts to destroy Marie's future by making her feel bad for making progress in her life. Her methods are clearly covert since she is so sneaky about it that her own sister does not seem to notice them. Moreover, since she is so focused on her success in school and values her grades even when her mental health is declining, she is obviously a cerebral narcissist.

The cause of Anne's NPD seems clear, given her history. She is mourning the childhood she had before her father left. If Marie heard the fights, then Anne probably did as well. She was even younger than her sister at the time of the divorce, so she had less time to become secure in her identity and let her personality develop. Her failure to make friends in her new school also did not help to make her more secure, and she may have lost her ability to empathize after stressing over her peer's opinions for too long. Her heart hardened itself in self-defense, and she started painting herself as a constant victim of even small offenses as a means of gaining sympathy and shifting blame.

From their father's interactions with their mother, it seems as though he might be suffering from some type of personality disorder as well. In particular, he may be histrionic or paranoid. Histrionic personality disorder is defined by a series of violent outbursts as an attempt to gain attention. He might have been accusing his wife of different wrongs as an effort to get her eyes on him, even if it was in a negative fashion.

Paranoid personality disorder is defined in its name. Someone who has PPD has a series of paranoid delusions about their environment and the people around them. And as we learned in chapter 4, both of these disorders have a strong connection with NPD in terms of inheritability. He likely passed the gene to both of his daughters, and it triggered a disorder in his more delicate, younger child.

Malignant Narcissist

In Northern California, a small family of four lives in a humble home—Hope (the mother) and her three children (Al, Melissa, and Theo). They've lived in the area for their whole lives and are fairly well-established. Hope is a writer at a law firm, Al is going to college in a few months, and Melissa and Theo are doing their best in school so they can follow in their oldest brother's footsteps.

Secretly, neither child wants to be anything like Al. Al's personality started going downhill when he was in fourth grade. He had some sort of fallout with his friends at the time, and although no one remembers what it was about, it was probably petty and didn't mean much in the grand scheme of things. What could a bunch of fourth graders be doing that would warrant so much drama? However the fight started, it ended with his former friends starting a rumor about him, him getting upset, and a few weeks later, him punching one of them in the jaw.

Sure, Al had some anger issues before then, but it was not anything outside of the realm of normalcy for a young child, and it certainly was never directed toward his younger siblings. However, after that display of anger, he just could not seem to stop. Most of it was directed toward Theo, but only because mom was more lenient with them. She would always say, "Boys will be boys." She would be more upset if he hurt Melissa, her little girl. Unfortunately for Melissa, she still was not free from the constant humiliation, belittling, and gaslighting that Al seemed to spew nonstop.

Frankly, he is not the easiest to be around. He only talks about himself and his day, and if you try to talk about yourself, he appears visibly bored and brings the conversation back around to himself very quickly. The stuff he talks about can be a bit uncomfortable, too. He is a handsome teenager, so he picks up a lot of girls around school and is eager to tell you about each and every one of them. If he is not talking about that, he is talking about his fitness routine, which neither sibling finds very interesting. He gets angry if you do not listen, though, so it is best to sit quietly and let him talk.

The fights usually started when either sibling dared to disagree with him or engage in some light teasing. Insulting him was a bad idea, even if it was intended as a joke, and it usually resulted in some sort of revenge scheme that involved lying to mom and getting somebody in trouble. Mom would make excuses for Al and say that he is just sensitive, but something felt wrong to Melissa and Theo. Al was not doing this because he was legitimately offended; he did it because he wanted some excuse to abuse his siblings. He got some type of enjoyment from this.

Melissa and Theo had their suspicions that Al had NPD and decided to do some research, which eventually led them to ask their mother about their father. They learned that she kicked out their dad when Al was only an infant because she noticed that he abused him and she was not about to sit aside and let it happen. The younger two were born to a different man whom she divorced because he cheated on her. She wouldn't admit that this had something to do with Al's behavior, but the children knew that this trauma certainly affected him in some way.

So although the siblings are glad that Al will be going away to college, they are worried about how he will do. Will he get in trouble with the university? Will he bully the other students or his roommates? How will he be when he comes home for vacation? Will the new-found freedom make him better or worse?

Analysis

Al is not the most violent malignant narcissist we have looked at so far, but his sadism gives him away. Ever since he was young, he engaged in violent behaviors and seemed to think of himself as better than others, which he made clear in his actions. He is also slightly manipulative, as seen in the way his mother makes excuses for him and often allows him to bully Theo. However, all in all, his methods are very overt.

Since Al places a lot of value on the girls he dates and on his body, it is easy to peg him as a somatic narcissist. He probably does not care much about any of the girls he takes to bed, but he uses them as bragging pieces to prove his sexual prowess anyway. He also struggles to empathize with others in conversation, so he would rather talk about something that is more relevant to him: his personal fitness. It seems that his false self mostly consists of sex, the gym, and anger. He is trying to portray himself as the ultimate man—the combination of all stereotypically masculine traits.

The information that Melissa and Theo learned about their father is very helpful in sorting out the full context of the situation. Although they believed that the incident in fourth grade was when everything started, it seemed as though Al had been subjected to abuse that the other two siblings were not. Also, since he has a different father than the other two, there is a high chance that his genes were different and made him more susceptible to developing NPD. The disorder was there, waiting, and arose when Al realized that getting angry and putting other people down was an easy way to make him feel better about himself.

Chapter 6:

Identify and Disarm the Narcissist to Protect Yourself

Abuse comes in many shapes, sizes, and forms. It is affected by various factors, including the personality of the abuser, the weaknesses of the victim, and the living arrangements between them. Ultimately, most kinds of abuse come down to a single desire of the perpetrator: a need for control.

For the narcissist, controlling someone means keeping them in an "inferior" position. The narcissist will define for themselves what it means to be superior or inferior and will attempt to force those roles onto both themselves and those around them through manipulation, lies, or even violence. The abuse of a narcissist is unique from other types, so there is no surprise that we have a term to describe its nature: narcissistic abuse.

What Is Narcissistic Abuse?

We use the term narcissistic abuse to refer to any abuse in which the perpetrator is a narcissist. An individual who inflicts narcissistic abuse may not have a diagnosis, but they must fulfill the major requirements of the diagnosis or at least have a number of narcissistic traits in order for the term to be used.

People who have suffered narcissistic abuse tend to experience a unique list of hardships, and these symptoms are often referred to as narcissistic abuse syndrome. After an individual has lived with a narcissist for a long time, they are extremely likely to develop a number of symptoms that they may struggle with even when the narcissistic abuse itself has ended. For instance, an individual may remain hyper-vigilant, have a number of intrusive/invasive thoughts, have flashbacks, feel detached from others, and have a hard time trusting others. They may have also fallen for a number of the narcissist's gaslighting techniques, which make them think that they are the narcissist, that the narcissist is the only person who cares about them, and that they may also have a positive opinion of their abuser (Rosglas Recovery, 2019).

If you are suffering from narcissistic abuse syndrome, a number of these symptoms may sound very familiar. Perhaps you often question whether or not you are the truly narcissistic sibling, or perhaps you have low self-esteem and struggle to trust others after spending the first few decades of your life with a volatile or sadistic narcissist. However your sibling makes you feel, your pain is valid and understandable, and it is shared by many others.

The exact nature of the abuse you endured may differ based on the tactics your sibling used. Let us take a look at some of the specific outbreaks of violence that may have been enacted on you.

Types of Abuse

What do you typically picture when you hear the word "abuse"? Give yourself a second to let a few images enter your mind. Do you picture a domestic abuse case where a husband is hitting his wife? Do you picture parental abuse where a parent deals a harsh punishment to their child? Are you only imagining physical abuse, or do you also imagine a verbal assault?

If you are like the majority of the population, you probably first imagined domestic abuse. The perpetrator is probably the husband. His wife is his victim, and he is probably using some sort of physical violence. He may also be yelling, swearing, and calling her a number of degrading words. Unfortunately, this type of abuse is very common, but it is not the only form of abuse. Sometimes, people are hurt in quiet, subtle ways, and their pain is not any less distressing, any less difficult to navigate, or any easier to heal from. Your sibling may have hurt you in a number of different ways that can all substitute abuse, so don't discount all of the ways in which you might be hurting.

Narcissistic abuse may involve a variety of abuse tactics. According to Lancer (2017), these are a few examples of how abuse can look:

- **Physical:** This is the type of abuse that most people picture. It can include hitting, slapping, pulling your hair, throwing objects, restraining you, or anything else that involves your body. Destroying your property also falls in the realm of physical abuse.

- **Verbal:** We all say things that we regret sometimes, but an abuser will often use words as a means of putting people down on purpose in order to get their way. Verbal abuse entails bullying, blaming, shaming, threatening, and even interrupting.

- **Neglect:** If your sibling is responsible for providing a certain need of yours and purposefully denies you of it, they are neglectful. Neglect also means placing the victim in a dangerous situation, which is sometimes referred to as "endangerment."

- **Privacy invasion:** Prying into someone's personal emails, texts, mail, and belongings is not just rude; it is abuse. This form of abuse comes into play when you attempt to set a boundary with an abuser and that boundary is disrespected.

- **Financial abuse:** Money runs the world, and it is also an easy way to control someone if it is placed in the wrong hands. Financial abuse is fairly common and involves denying a person's access to their money, spending someone's money without permission, selling personal property, or otherwise using money as a means of keeping someone under control.

- **Isolation:** This form of abuse can be common in romantic relationships. An abusive partner may restrict their significant other from seeing their friends and family. They limit their access to the outside world. If your sibling attempts to keep you from talking to certain people, they want you to feel isolated.

- **Gaslighting:** We have discussed gaslighting a few times already, and it does qualify as a form of abuse. If someone is gaslighting you, they will try to convince you that you are crazy, that your sense of reality is skewed, or that you are simply incompetent.

- **Withholding:** This is a much lesser-known form of abuse. When an abuser withholds something their victim wants or needs until the victim acts the way they want, it falls under this category.

- **Slander:** Slander involves spreading lies or rumors about a person in an attempt to ruin their reputation or sabotage their social lives. Destroying a person's intrapersonal relationships is a cruel way to get full control of them.
- **Competition:** Competition is a normal part of many brotherhoods and sisterhoods, but sometimes it can be taken too far. A narcissist may use competition as a way of making themselves look better than you.
- **Emotional blackmail:** Blackmail involves the use of threats, warnings, and intimidation as a way of getting someone to cooperate. Although it involves a lot of verbal abuse, it falls under a different category because of the inclusion of action.

The Cycle of Abuse

A narcissist's behavior can seem erratic and unpredictable, especially in individuals with more violent tendencies. The people around them are left feeling like they are walking on their tiptoes, carefully avoiding anything that could offend the narcissist in the hopes of keeping things calm and civil. As the sibling of a narcissist, you understand this better than anyone, but you may have already noticed a pattern in your sibling's moods.

Your observations are accurate. Like most abusers, narcissists follow a cyclical pattern of behaviors. Each time through the cycle may look different in drastic ways, but the narcissist's mindset and motivation behind their actions remain the same. Christine Hammond, MS, describes four different steps in the cycle of narcissistic abuse in her article "The Narcissistic Cycle of Abuse Among Siblings."

You may be wondering why it is worthwhile to understand the cycle of narcissistic abuse. If the aim is to escape, what is the point of analyzing your sibling's mindset or trying to understand what they are doing? Isn't empathizing with them a bit counter-intuitive? Well, the end goal is not exactly empathy. It is understanding. When you come to recognize the cycle of abuse, you will be able to break free of it. You can predict future confrontations, make sense of past arguments, and learn to keep yourself safe by implementing techniques such as going no contact and setting new boundaries. Knowing this cycle and where you currently stand will be helpful as you begin to defend yourself.

Step 1: The Narcissist Feels Threatened

In the first step of the cycle, the narcissist feels threatened by an upsetting event. The exact nature of the threat itself is likely to differ with each new rotation through the cycle. Perhaps your sibling experiences some sort of personal trigger, is embarrassed in public, becomes jealous of someone else's success, or feels disrespected in some way. The trigger may not be obvious at first, especially if your sibling is a vulnerable narcissist who may hide their emotions in an attempt to manipulate, but the trigger will exist regardless. Thankfully, however, the exact nature of the threat will not need to be identified in order for you to understand and predict the rest of the cycle. In fact, the next few steps may give you a hint as to what threatens your sibling in the first place.

If you want to identify the trigger, you can start by looking back at your sibling's past behaviors and examining what they usually get upset by. Most narcissists will obsess over a particular type of threat. If they are somatic, they will obsess over their appearance, sex life, sexual partners, or perhaps workouts. They may feel threatened by someone whom they perceive as more beautiful than themselves or someone who has obtained a sexual partner that they desire. If the narcissist is cerebral, they will be more focused on matters of the mind. They are susceptible to being jealous of people who are successful, intelligent, or anything else that shows that they have a superior mind. Regardless of whether your sibling is somatic or cerebral, they may have a number of different triggers related to their past, insecurities, or general personality.

Step 2: The Narcissist Abuses Others

After the narcissist feels threatened, they will act out and abuse whoever or whatever they perceive to be the offending party. The way in which they act out will vary depending on a number of factors, including the type of narcissist they are, the methods of abuse they prefer, and what they feel the weakness of their victim is. For instance, an overt narcissist may be very upfront about the abuse and tend to be physical or verbal. They often engage in emotional blackmail. A covert narcissist, however, may engage in some sort of self-sacrificing behavior that they can later use to paint their victim as the bad guy. A malicious narcissist is the most likely to be physical, and a vulnerable narcissist will be the most manipulative and sneaky.

Ultimately, the narcissist's goal during this phase is to get their victim to act in self-defense. They want to get a reaction out of you, whether that means insulting them back, hitting, or calling them out on manipulative behavior. This stage of the cycle can last for as long as it takes for someone to get fed up with the abuse and take action.

Step 3: The Narcissist Becomes the Victim

During this step, the narcissist will twist the story to appear to be the victim. In many cases, this is where the dissociation and confabulation associated with the false self come in. The narcissist has fully convinced themselves that they are the victim in this situation because they can't imagine a reality where they could be the abuser. They will be determined to convince others of this delusion as well. This is the stage where gaslighting, guilting, and shaming occur.

In the narcissist's best-case scenario, their victim will happily take the blame and agree to the narcissist's warped version of reality. To them, this is as good as an admission of inferiority, and it usually leaves the victim feeling ashamed and frustrated. In some cases, the narcissist may be eager to tell others about how they were "victimized" in order to get more people on their side.

Step 4: The Narcissist Is Empowered

After they have established themselves as the victim, the narcissist believes they have won. They will feel justified and validated in their belief that they are the better sibling, and they will feel that they have sufficiently proven that idea to others. Their victim has unknowingly fed their ego and made their warped reality more solidified in their minds by agreeing with it, even though the victim was well-intentioned and simply wanted to keep the peace.

Also, the narcissist will remember this cycle and keep it in the back of their mind the next time they are feeling threatened. They will remember which abuse methods elicited a reaction from their victim, and they may even talk about this cycle during the next one. When they are painting themselves as the victim next time, they may mention how they were abused during the last cycle and how it is happening again. This makes their gaslighting efforts even easier. After several cycles, the narcissist will have their victim under their thumb, completely buying into their false reality.

Keeping Yourself Safe

The No-Contact Rule

You have had enough. You have had your heart broken thousands of times. You have lost years of your childhood to shame and manipulation, and you feel ready to start a new chapter of your life. You are ready to stand up to your sibling, and you have determined that you would be much more successful if your sibling was no longer a major factor.

If that sounds like you, you may be ready to start a no-contract rule. The name explains it all: through this rule, you either temporarily or permanently cease communication with someone who affects you in a negative way. In this case, the negative influence is your sibling, but the no-contact rule is used in all sorts of toxic relationships. You can use the time away from your sibling to let yourself heal and start a new life before you attempt to interact with them again, or you can make it into a permanent rule in order to ensure that the trauma does not happen again. Natasha Adamo, the author of *Win Your Breakup*, sees no-contact as a period of self-care:

"I define the no-contact rule as a way to resurrect your backbone, build unconditional confidence ... and attain classy revenge without having to disembark from the dignity, standards, and self-respect that you are trying to rebuild" (Adamo, 2020).

Adamo also emphasizes that, despite being an extremely effective means of promoting healing, the no-contact rule has to be done with the right mindset if it is going to be helpful in any lasting way. You cannot go no contact to see how your sibling reacts, and you cannot use it to be spiteful. You must approach the no-contact rule as a means of protecting yourself from physical and psychological attacks so that you can grow as a person.

The beauty of going no contact is this: You don't owe your sibling an explanation. You don't need to spell out the reasons why you want to go no contact. You don't have to beg them to empathize, and you don't need to defend yourself. You can simply state that you need to stop communicating, and then you can go ahead and block the narcissist on social media. They may still send you texts or attempt to break the no-contact rule in other ways, but you can (and should!) simply ignore their pursuit at re-establishing a relationship. If contact is absolutely necessary, keep the conversation polite, but end it quickly. Say whatever needs to be said, and then leave (Adamo, 2020).

It is also entirely your decision whether or not you would like to explain your motives to your parents and other family members. Giving them your point of view may help to keep them on good terms with you and prevent the narcissist from twisting the truth, but it is not necessary if you would rather keep this decision to yourself.

Maintaining no contact can be difficult. People with narcissistic abuse syndrome are used to constant belittlement, manipulation, and pain, so they might struggle when that way of life is changed. Andrea Schneider, LCSW, explains that "some [people with narcissistic abuse syndrome] have likened the experience to like coming off a drug; it is so painful to go through the traumatic grief work in being abandoned that these feelings are akin to withdrawals" (Adamo, 2020). However, if the victim is able to endure this withdrawal and enforces the no-contact rule, they will quickly see improvement in their mental health.

Setting Boundaries

Although experts agree that going no contact is the best-case scenario for anyone with narcissistic abuse syndrome, I know that it is not always a realistic option. Many of us still live under the same roof as our siblings, so some sense of communication needs to exist for the household to run smoothly. Still, it is possible to create boundaries with your sibling in order to give yourself a bit of space to heal, create yourself, and gain back some confidence.

First, take a few moments to decide what you need in order to feel safer at home. Perhaps you can use your room as a safe space, have certain devices that you contact friends with, or even engage in personal hobbies that can get you out of the house and give you some distance. Consider the ways in which your sibling complicates those securities. Do they enter your room when you are trying to escape? Do they participate in your hobbies when you would prefer to create some space between the two of you? Do they constantly send angry texts to your phone? Also, consider whether or not your sibling respects your physical boundaries. Do they touch you when you would rather be left alone?

After establishing the areas of your life where you could use a bit of space, you will need to state your intentions clearly. Similar to creating a no-contact rule, you should not feel pressured to explain your intentions to your sibling if you would rather save yourself the trouble. You can simply state, "Don't text me after 7:00 p.m.," or any other boundary you would like to set.

If your sibling does not respect the boundary, try restating it to see if that helps. We are all human and can be forgetful at times, so it is possible that your sibling has simply forgotten that the boundary exists. If that still does not work, try giving a reason alongside the statement. Your reason can be honest if you feel safe discussing that with your sibling, but you can also come up with an excuse if you need to. Returning to our earlier example, you could state, "I asked you not to text me after 7:00 p.m. because I am struggling to focus on schoolwork and need some time away from my phone." After that, simply stop answering your phone. Giving someone the silent treatment can be hard, but if it can help your mental health, it is worth the effort.

Don't Take Things Personally

Even if you go no contact or successfully set boundaries with your sibling, chances are pretty high that you will still be interacting with them in some way during various points of your life. There will always be weddings, funerals, family gatherings, and other events that will bring the two of you together. When that happens, you will need a few techniques up your sleeve to help keep you safe from their abuse.

In moments where I am forced to interact with the narcissist in my life, I find it helpful to remember everything I have learned about NPD and remind myself that there is a reason why a narcissist acts how they do. A narcissist, like anyone else with a mental illness or personality disorder, experiences reality in a different way. They hide behind a false self, bury their insecurities, and use others as a means of raising their own self-esteem. A narcissistic sibling would abuse anyone else they spent a lot of time with; it is not exclusive to you. When you learn to stop taking their insults personally, you can emotionally distance yourself from the abuse and lessen its hold on your life. You have done nothing wrong, so you don't need to feel any shame or guilt.

Give yourself plenty of self-care before and after interacting with your sibling, and try to keep things in perspective. Your sibling has a personality disorder that leads them to behave a certain way, and although it can be extremely hurtful, it is beyond the narcissist's control. It does not reflect you, your character, or your worth. Keep doing your own thing and allow your sibling's toxic ideas to fall to the side. This is certainly easier said than done, but it will become easier with time.

Ignore the Taunts

Even if you can't physically distance yourself from your sibling, you can still emotionally distance yourself. You will remember from the cycle of abuse that the transition between step 1 and step 2 depends on the victim lashing out in some way after suffering abuse from the narcissist, so you have a lot of control during that point of the cycle.

Instead of getting angry when your sibling confronts you, take a moment to yourself and try to relax. You can use any number of grounding techniques, such as counting to 10, taking a few deep breaths, or making a list of objects in your mind. You can also try distracting yourself by engaging in a hobby, listening to music, or doing anything that will calm you down.

I understand that it is frustrating to have to rein in your own emotions when you are the victim, but it is important to remember that staying calm will keep you safe. You simply have to outlast the narcissist and make them give up on getting a reaction out of you. Doing so will completely dismantle the cycle and will make your sibling less likely to abuse you in the future.

Stop Blaming Yourself

Letting go of the guilt and shame that you hold will not only improve your mental health but also help ultimately stop the abuse. During step 3 of the abuse cycle, the narcissist tries to convince their victim to accept the blame and agree with the narcissist's reality, so ceasing to accept blame is an easy way to throw off the narcissist.

The key to doing this successfully is to not get angry. Arguing with the narcissist is not going to be productive, and they will simply use your anger as ammunition to paint you as the villain. Instead, excuse yourself from the conversation. Refuse to participate in any conversation where you are being slandered, and be sure to appear self-assured and untouched by the insults. If the narcissist is not able to knock you down, they will eventually stop trying.

All in all, remember that everything the narcissist does only speaks poorly of them. They may have everyone fooled, and they may have told others that you are a terrible person. However, so long as you know that you are doing the right thing, you can live a healthy, productive life. E. B. Johnson (2020) says it best:

> The problems that this person has are not your fault, and they are (ultimately) not your problem. Having compassion for someone is not the same as taking on their pain and issues for yourself. Detach from their behavior and understanding that all this lashing out has everything to do with them and very little to do with you.

Success Stories

When I read stories about people successfully implementing a no-contact rule, establishing new boundaries, or simply caring less about their narcissistic sibling's opinions, I am filled with hope. Everyone's lives are different, and no experience is quite like yours, but if someone else can do it, so can you!

Example 1: Hard-Won Victory

This touching story was shared on Reddit in December 2020. This user was raised by a Catholic family in America's South, and his narcissistic parents did not approve when he came out as gay. He was abused before, but it increased tenfold after that. He was constantly told that he was lazy and worthless, and they did nothing to intervene when he was sexually abused. He ended up meeting a partner online and moved out to live with him, which was a wonderful arrangement for both of them for a long time.

However, narcissists are sneaky and determined. They contacted one of his friends to try to get contact information, and when that did not work, they lied about his mother's health going downhill as a trick to get him to visit. However, he reports that he is now going no contact with both parents and has been living a lot happier since then.

Example 2: Moving Forward

Another Reddit user shared an update about her breakup with a narcissist. They used to spend New Year's Eve together, as many couples do, so her first time facing the holiday without him was rough. She remembers locking herself in her room and crying over him. It was not a good start to her year, but thankfully, she has been doing better since then. This is what she has to say, and she hopes that her success can bring hope to others in a similar situation:

> Today I am at peace. I made it through the other side, where I can see with more clarity that I dodged a lifetime of anxiety and misery. I am going through difficult times in my life ... but I genuinely feel grateful I do not have this ache in my heart anymore over him that used to make me sob for nights on end.

Although it often takes a lot of healing to recover from a narcissist's abuse, it is possible to move on.

Example 3: To Block or Not?

When going no contact with a narcissist, our modern world offers some unique challenges. Each individual has to decide for themselves whether they want to block their abuser on social media and whether they want to keep their phone number available at all. There is no right or wrong answer to this dilemma because it will vary a lot based on your personal circumstances. Reddit user Tnstone also had to navigate this, and his answer was to block all methods of contact with his narcissistic sister.

At first, he only blocked her on social media. He wanted to keep his sibling's phone number in case of any emergencies with their nieces and nephews, but she took advantage of that small window of contact and sent plenty of manipulative messages. She was angry about being blocked on social media, tried to prove her innocence, and instructed the Redditor to go to therapy "because something is obviously wrong with you." In reality, the Redditor had already gone to therapy, and the therapist was assisting with the no-contact rule.

In the end, the narcissist's number was blocked from his phone entirely. He made an arrangement with their mother that she would mediate between the two siblings in case of an emergency so that they wouldn't have to interact directly, and it has been going well.

Chapter 7:

Healing From a

Narcissist's Abuse

Escaping from a narcissist's grasp means more than simply stopping the abuse or creating distance between the two of you; it also means moving forward with your life. Ultimately, your aim is to create a better life for yourself and recover from everything you have been put through. No matter what degree of abuse you endured, you deserve to take the time to care for yourself and heal before you begin the rest of your life. As you will learn in this chapter, a bit of self-care can also prevent mental blockages years down the line, so you will be doing yourself a huge favor by slowing down and mending your mental wounds.

In this chapter, we will take a look at C-PTSD, or complex post-traumatic stress disorder, which is commonly caused by narcissistic abuse. We will examine its symptoms and clinical treatments before looking at some self-care techniques that you can use to lessen the symptoms on your own.

What Is C-PTSD?

Most people have encountered the term PTSD (post-traumatic stress disorder) at some point in their lives. They probably associate it with war veterans who struggle with the violence they endured while serving in the military and who have frequent flashbacks to that time. Those veterans are pulled back into the past by the sound of a firework, by someone moving too quickly, or other personal triggers, making their lives difficult to live. You also may have heard of people developing PTSD after a traumatic event, such as a car crash, the 9/11 explosion, an assault, and more. Either way, people who struggle with moving forward after a single traumatic experience may have developed PTSD.

However, trauma comes in many forms, and it is sometimes drawn out over multiple years. Someone who is abused by their spouse may not be traumatized by a single night of abuse but is weighed down by years and years of mistreatment. That sort of trauma sometimes causes a person to develop complex post-traumatic stress disorder (C-PTSD).

In Madeline Kennedy's medically reviewed article about post-traumatic stress for Insider.com, she describes the difference between PTSD and C-PTSD as follows: "PTSD usually occurs after a singular traumatic event, while C-PTSD is associated with repeated trauma" (Kennedy, 2020).

As someone who has been living with a narcissist as a sibling, you may be more likely to experience C-PTSD than traditional PTSD. It would be worthwhile for you to read through the symptoms and see if anything clicks for you, as it will help you to recognize the nature of your trauma and begin to heal from it.

Symptoms of C-PTSD

PTSD and C-PTSD are very similar, but people with C-PTSD will experience a few extra symptoms on top of those of PTSD. David Berle, a clinical psychologist and a professor of psychology at the University of Technology Sydney, says that "people with C-PTSD typically experience the full gamut of PTSD symptoms," even though the symptoms may manifest in slightly different ways. For instance, people with both PTSD and C-PTSD are likely to have the following signs:

- Reliving trauma
- Avoiding people, situations, or places that remind them of their trauma
- Mood fluctuations that did not exist prior to the trauma
- Feeling on edge, irritable, jumpy, or easily frightened

Although people with C-PTSD do relive their trauma, they may not realize when a flashback is occurring. In these emotional flashbacks, a person re-experiences some of the strong emotions they had during their trauma, such as shame, fear, sadness, or embarrassment. They may also react to events happening in the present in the same way that they felt during their trauma, as though the new experience was the same as their trauma. Most people with C-PTSD do not realize that this is another type of flashback, so they may not even know that it is related to their trauma (Mind, 2017).

On top of the previous list of symptoms, C-PTSD sufferers are more likely to experience the following:

- Difficulties maintaining relationships
- Difficulties managing emotions
- Feelings of shame, self-hate, or worthlessness
- Physical symptoms, such as headaches, stomach pains, or chest pains
- Suicidal thoughts

If those symptoms sound familiar, it is likely that you have C-PTSD or are at least dealing with a lot of long-term trauma. In the next chapter, we will talk a bit more about how professional therapy can benefit both you and your sibling, but first, I will take a moment to talk about what it means to treat C-PTSD in a clinical setting.

Treating C-PTSD

In general, a therapist will aim to help you process your trauma in a safe environment. They are trained to help deal with any panic that arises during that process so that you can stay focused on making progress instead of being overwhelmed by fear or shame. Although PTSD typically takes about 8–12 therapy sessions to get under control, C-PTSD takes much longer: about six months of consistent sessions. This is because victims of C-PTSD developed more habits to defend themselves from constant abuse, so it takes more time to replace those habits with healthy, productive ones instead.

Although there are not any medications specific to C-PTSD, your therapist may recommend some of the medicines commonly used for PTSD, such as antidepressants (e.g., Zoloft and Paxil) or anti-anxiety medications (e.g., Klonopin). A therapist would help you overcome the instincts that lead you to isolate yourself, protect yourself, and constantly look for danger. Treating C-PTSD typically also involves a lot of skill-learning. Since the trauma was prolonged and may have started in early childhood, an individual with the diagnosis may not have the skills (such as self-care) to fight negative feelings (Kennedy, 2020). For the remainder of this chapter, we will address some of the skills you can teach yourself even without therapy.

Some studies have even shown that mindfulness-based stress relief (MBSR) has great benefits for those who suffer from trauma. MBSR is an eight-week program that uses the practice of mindfulness, a form of meditation that helps ground a person in their present surroundings, to help improve a person's mindset and move on from symptoms of depression, anxiety, stress, and more. There is also positive evidence of acupuncture being helpful for those who need to cope with trauma. A physician may recommend that you engage in one of these activities, or you can pursue them on your own (Trauma Recovery, 2013). You can even seek MBSR for free or for a low cost online.

Recognize and Change Your Mindset

Julie L. Hall is a narcissist abuse recovery coach. She specializes in helping people who have been targeted by narcissists. She has worked with many clients who are dealing with the same situation that you are in, and she has a fundamental understanding of what it means to be a narcissist and how that can affect the narcissist's family, peers, and friends.

Hall (2019) shares six insights to Psychology.com for people who have begun the healing process so that they can recognize and change their mindset from fearful and damaged to prosperous.

1. Realize that this is a large, systemic problem. Hall's clients tend to place blame. They either blame themselves for their own abuse or become angry with the narcissist in their lives. Although this is an understandable reaction, there is never a single individual or situation to blame for a narcissist's behavior. As you have learned in this text, it takes multiple factors for a narcissist to be created, and many people usually buy into the narcissist's false self. Rather than placing blame, try to step back and understand the situation as a whole.

2. Denial feels euphoric, but it is ultimately harmful. At the start of your recovery, you may be in denial of how much you are hurting, or perhaps you deny that your sibling has NPD at all. Denial helps us to feel better in the short term, but it will cause tons of problems if you hold on to it. Eliminating that denial is often the first and hardest step of recovery, and it is very necessary. Give yourself some space to look inside of yourself, examine the truth, and feel the full force of it.

3. Understand the strength of NPD. Hall emphasizes that people with empathy have a very hard time understanding NPD and usually overestimate a narcissist's ability to love others. She states that a narcissist only cares about the services and goods that a person can provide, not specifically the person, so even your good memories with the narcissist are not evidence of love as we understand it. Do not let those good memories get in the way of your ability to move on.

4. Let yourself feel everything that you need to feel. Grief finds a way of affecting us, even if we try to bottle it away. It is absolutely key to allow yourself to mourn everything that you need to mourn, whether it is the childhood you missed out on, the sibling you wish you had, the sibling you thought you knew, or the other relationships that your sibling sabotaged. It is tempting to try distracting yourself from that pain, but facing that grief and letting yourself feel it in its full force will save you a lot of trouble years down the line.

5. Recognize that you are traumatized. Now is not the time to act tough. You have encountered constant belittling and have been made to question your own sanity and self-worth. In order to address your symptoms, you must first realize that the symptoms exist and that you can benefit from recovery.

6. Know that healing is possible. Everyone is capable of healing, just like everyone is capable of hurting. After recognizing your mindset, fighting your denial, and letting yourself feel the full extent of your grief and injury, you can make a full recovery and become a happier, more fulfilled person. The rest of your life is not determined by the people who lived with you for the first few decades, and you will be surprised at everything you can achieve in the next few years. Don't give up!

Self-Care

Even if you cannot pursue professional therapy or get a diagnosis, you can still help yourself heal from trauma on your own. When a person takes the time to heal themselves, we call it "self-care." There are many different styles of self-care that will be more or less effective, depending on the individual. Most of the time, they involve adding something new to your daily life that will improve your quality of life in some way, but sometimes self-care means securing a mundane activity in your schedule that you are struggling with. For instance, if you have been too depressed to shower for the last week, starting to shower every morning will help you feel refreshed and ready for the day.

The most important thing to remember when performing self-care is that it is not selfish. You are not "pampering" yourself. You are not becoming "spoiled," and you certainly are not being a narcissist. Instead, you are taking the time to become the best version of yourself that you can be. Healing from your trauma will improve your life in ways that you may not even think of, so it will be worthwhile to take the time out of your day to perform a self-care activity or two.

I have provided a list of self-care activities from Beauty After Bruises, a non-profit organization that is dedicated to helping people who are suffering from C-PTSD by offering grants, advice, and other support. Their list is specifically designed for survivors of trauma and abuse, especially those with complex traumas that can be more complicated to sort through in normal therapy. These activities are split into three different categories: easy, moderate, and difficult.

The easy techniques will only take a few minutes and don't require many materials, but they also have the smallest impact on your mental health. The moderate activities are more effective but will also take more time. The difficult activities are long-term commitments that will help you develop new habits and create a new mindset. You may find it easier to start with the shorter activities, but if you feel ready to tackle the hard ones, go for it!

Also, remember that not all of these activities are going to work for you. In fact, you may even find that some of them make you even more stressed or are simply ineffective at pulling your mind away from your trauma. If that happens, don't worry. Just try another activity on the list and see how it goes.

Easy Self-Care Activities

- Take 10-minute breaks from whatever you are doing. Whether you have been working on homework for hours, doing chores, or even scrolling social media, try taking a 10-minute break every hour to sit back and relax. You can use this time to meditate or simply make yourself a glass of tea and savor it. You can even head outside for some sunshine!

- Take a nap. Plenty of trauma survivors suffer from a lack of rest, so feel free to let yourself make up for your lost z's by snoozing during the day. Let yourself nap in a space where you feel safe and can let your guard down for a while.

- Watch reruns of your favorite show, sports games, or YouTube videos. You already know the outcome, plot twists, and jokes, so a rewatch can give you a stress-free watching experience.

- Text a friend. You don't need to talk about your trauma if you don't want to. Simply chatting with a loved one about your day or the weather can be a great mood lifter.

- Make a list of 10 things you like about yourself, 10 accomplishments you have made over the last year, or 10 things you are grateful for. Lists like those are a great way to get your mind on to some positive things in your life.

- Repeat some personal affirmations. Affirmations are "I am" statements that can help us reprogram our brains. You can say them out loud, in your head, or in front of a mirror. You can also try writing them down. Try affirmations like "I am worthy," "I am good enough," and "I am innocent."

- Take your medications as needed. It is easy to fall behind on prescriptions or think you are not feeling "bad enough" for your PRNs. If you need them, give yourself permission to take them.

- Use a weighted blanket, weighted lap mat, or weighted vest. Many people who struggle with anxious thoughts find that they feel safer and more secure under something heavy. If you don't have any of those items, try applying pressure on your body with your hands, or put a book under your laptop for some extra weight. You can even try the thickest blanket in your house to see if it adds some extra security.

- Take a photoshoot with yourself. Especially if your sibling is somatic, you may have been convinced that you are not beautiful. Put on your favorite outfit and snap a few pics!

Moderate Self-Care Activities

- Read a book. You can reread an old favorite, start a new story, or choose a nonfiction novel and learn something new. Books are a great way to distract the mind and help you realize that there is more to life than whatever situation you are in or what you have lived through.
- Examine your calendar and see if there are any responsibilities that you can remove or ask someone else to complete. Doing this will help you clear more time for other self-care activities.
- Reach out to online support groups or hunt for in-person groups in your area. There are more people than you think who have experienced the same things as you, and talking to them may be helpful.

- Give yourself a spa day. Make a nice bath, light some candles, and use all of your favorite skin care products. If you like to shave your body hair or paint your nails, a spa day would be a great time to do that, too!
- Stretch, do some yoga, or go for a walk. Simple activities like that can help reconnect you to your body and put you in the present.
- Wear your favorite clothes, even if they are not socially acceptable. Wearing things you actually like does not hurt anyone, but it can help you immensely.
- Clean your living space. We don't always notice it, but living in a chaotic space makes our minds more chaotic, too. Taking 30 minutes to clean your room or home can make a big difference.
- Watch something that you know will make you cry. Releasing emotions helps us feel free, even if you are crying over a fictional character.
- Go for a long drive. Put on some of your favorite music, roll the windows down, and see what you can find!
- Buy yourself something nice. Retail therapy is real, and although it should not be done too often, it feels great to enjoy something new that you really want. Make sure that it is not a basic necessity; it should be something extra that will spice up your day.

Difficult Self-Care Activities

- Start a journal. Although journaling is on the top of most self-care lists, no one seems to admit how hard it is to keep and maintain a journal. However, in spite of the difficulty, it can also be extremely rewarding. Try keeping a journal for a month and see if you like it!

- Enroll in a class. Is there anything you have always wanted to learn? Perhaps you are interested in whittling, coding, photography, or any other new hobby that requires a bit of skill. There are plenty of classes available online for various skills, and you can even search your area to see if there is anything you would be interested in.

- Attend a concert, play, show, or other performance. Life experiences like these can help us to feel motivated and passionate when we are disconnected and numb.

- Plan a mini-vacation, whether you do it alone or with friends. Pick a nearby city and drive there for a quick weekend stay!

- Get a new tattoo, haircut, piercing, or other body modification. Trauma sometimes causes us to feel like we are not in control of ourselves or our bodies, so getting a permanent (or semipermanent) change will remind you of the power you wield over yourself.

- Do some volunteer work. Your local animal shelter, soup kitchen, after-school programs, and other charities would be happy to have you. In turn, you will start to feel more fulfilled and see your worth even clearer.

- Connect with your spirituality or faith if it is applicable to you. Religion helps millions of people around the world make sense of the world, and pursuing something that helps you ignite your faith may make you feel stronger and less alone. Try attending a local service, reading some articles online, or sitting with a sacred text for a while.

- Set boundaries with other people in your life. We already talked about setting boundaries with your sibling, which is necessary, but take a moment to examine your life and see if you have been letting anyone else walk on you. Your sibling may have normalized that for you, so chances are pretty high that your other relationships could use some work as well.

Coping With Emotional Flashbacks

If you experience emotional flashbacks as a part of your C-PTSD or overall trauma response, then you know how difficult they can be to deal with. You overreact to small stressors, especially if they are related to things that your sibling used to do to you, and it makes you feel like a weak or over-emotional person. You may become overly defensive in the face of criticism, embarrassed of small weaknesses, or simply lose control of strong emotions when they arise. The people around you don't recognize that you are having a flashback, and you might not even know either, until you sit back and examine the incident.

Thankfully, you can use a number of techniques to make these flashbacks less frightening and detrimental. When you feel yourself becoming overly emotional in any situation, especially if you are getting the sense that you are overreacting or that the feeling is coming from a place of trauma, sit back and try one of these techniques recommended by Beauty After Bruises.

Grounding

The first thing you should do when you are having a trauma response is ground yourself. Grounding means becoming more aware of the present moment, your body, and the things around you when your mind is trying to pull you into the past. If you are ungrounded, the other techniques you try will not be as effective as they could be, so it is paramount to ensure that you are present and rooted before you proceed.

There are a lot of grounding techniques out there, and you may find that some work better for you than others. It may take some experimentation to find the best ones, and you won't want to experiment when you are actively having a flashback so that you can calm yourself as quickly as possible. Instead, try a few of these when you are calm and happy to see which ones are the most relaxing for you. You may even invent a technique that is not on this list, and that is okay too.

Here are some to get you started:

- De-trance yourself. If you tend to sway, bounce your leg, or make any other repetitive movement when you are having a flashback, slow the pattern to a stop and see if you can be still. You may also interrupt the movement with something drastically different, such as standing up so you can't bounce your leg anymore. If you have a tendency to stare into space, give yourself something to look at and focus on it, even if it is just a bird outside.
- Orient yourself and run through some basic facts. State your name, age, hometown, current location, and anything else that might feel good to you. You might even toss a few affirmations in, such as "I am safe."

- Engage your senses. If you often have flashbacks, you might want to carry mints with you so that you can pop one in your mouth once you become disoriented. The strong taste will help you stay rooted in the present. You can also take a sniff of a candle, some lotion, nearby food, or anything else that is strong.
- Safe touch can help a lot of people return to the moment. If you are alone, try running your fingertips over your arms, shoulders, and neck. You can touch some nearby textures, play with a zipper, or buy a fidget toy for yourself. If someone is helping you through the flashback and you are okay with having them touch you, you can ask to hold their hand or hug them.

Self-Talk

Once you are feeling more grounded, you can try a little bit of self-talk to ensure that you stay calm. Our inner monologues hold a lot of power and can affect the way we think about ourselves and others. It can also change our perception of the world around us and where we are, which we can use to our advantage. Much like the affirmations from earlier, you can say these aloud or in your head to change your thinking:

- "This is just a flashback. Nothing is hurting me in the present moment."

- "I am an adult now. My life is very different now than it used to be."
- "I have gone through this before, and I will get through it again."
- "This feeling is temporary."
- "I am in control."
- "I am worthy, and I am allowed to ask for help if I need it."

You can also try using more general affirmations, such as "I am amazing," "I am intelligent," or "I can do anything I put my mind to." Some people find that affirmations unrelated to the situation at hand provide a pleasant distraction without being disorienting, but others prefer to stay focused on what is right in front of them and how they are feeling in the moment.

Identify the Changing Times

This technique is very similar to self-talk, but it has a specific aim: to help you realize that your current situation is very different from the abuse you suffered. Taking the time to identify how you, your body, and the world around you have changed can be extremely comforting when facing a flashback. The exact nature of the change will vary a lot from person to person, so you may need to think about the sorts of things you might point out to yourself in a moment of panic. Here are a few examples so you can see exactly what I mean:

- Find a mirror and take a look at your body. Focus on how you look and how you have physically changed from how you used to be. Is your hair different? Have you lost or gained weight? Do you have wrinkles on your face now? Do you have any new tattoos or piercings? Even if you don't have a mirror, you can focus on how your hands have aged, how tall you are, and more.

- Look around the room at all of the technology. Do smartphones look different now, or do you have a new phone? Is your computer different?

- Identify the things that are yours that you did not have during the time of trauma. Try statements like "This is my house/apartment/dorm/room. These are my car keys. This is my driver's license."

- Think about where your sibling is currently located, their age, their relationship to you, and other things about them that may have changed.

- Watch a modern television show, listen to the newest music, or play your newest video game. While you do so, remind yourself that these things did not exist while you were being abused.

- Make a list of 10 positive things that have happened since the abuse.

Signs of Healing

Since progress can sometimes be very slow, we might feel like we are not improving at all. This is especially true if we are more introverted or isolated from the world and no one tells us that we are visibly recovering. Although this sounds like it is no big deal, it can actually be detrimental to a person's recovery. If you feel like you are not recovering at all, you might get very impatient with yourself, assume that your self-care is not working, and even cease your efforts because they feel pointless.

There are a few ways to avoid feeling this way. Many people find that journaling is helpful in this regard because you can look back at old entries and see how you have changed. Perhaps you can even include a mood tracker in your entries so that it is easier to flip through your journal quickly and see how you have been changing.

However, others don't enjoy journaling and will need some other ways to tell if they have been healing. According to Lampitt (2019), there are a number of signs that will tell you if you have been healing from your abuse, such as the following:

- You will start to feel lighter. Being under a narcissist's control keeps a person very tense, so when you have finally cut off that stress, your heart will feel like it is soaring.

- You may also feel physically lighter. It is very common for people to lose weight after cutting off a toxic relationship, especially if they are stress eaters or use food as a grounding technique. Consider keeping an eye on the scale to see if you have been losing a little weight, but be careful not to lose too much. Losing too much weight too quickly may be a sign of excessive grief.

- You will smile more. This one is a no-brainer, but many people don't notice how much they smile every day, so this sign goes over their heads. If you suddenly realize you are smiling (especially if there is no real reason for it), it is a strong sign that you are getting better.

- You feel a sense of relief and freedom. Since there are less intense stimuli in your life, you may even feel bored at first, but it is only because you are not used to having few stressors. It will feel better with time.

- Some of your physical symptoms will disappear, even if you did not realize the symptoms existed. Your headaches become less common, your stomach settles, and some of your muscle pains become less severe. If you have any chronic illnesses, you might notice fewer flare-ups.

- You will notice memory improvement. Your concentration and overall brain function will work great. Once your mind is no longer focused on survival, it will expand onto new and better things. You may also be seeing a positive change to your sleep schedule, which will help your mind flourish.
- Small, healthy habits may become more appealing. Your basic self-care will become easier to uphold, and you may develop an interest in some things you never thought about before, such as meditation, learning a new skill, exercising, and more.
- You will use escapism much less because the current world will become less frightening.
- You will think about your narcissistic sibling less. It may take some time for this to happen, but eventually, your life will develop beyond your narcissist, and you will have much better things to think about.

The Phases of Recovery

Alternatively, you may find it helpful to keep track of your current standing in the phases of recovery. TraumaRecovery.co defines three different phases of recovery after a person has experienced great trauma, whether that trauma aligns more closely with that of

PTSD or C-PTSD. Not everyone will follow these exact phases, but they are a good guideline for those who would like a probable timeline of their recovery. If you find that these phases don't resonate with you, don't stress! You can heal at your own pace and in your own way, and you don't need to stick to a schedule.

Phase 1: Safety and Stabilization

People recovering from immense trauma will feel unsafe in their bodies, surroundings, and relationships with others. This fear may manifest as trust issues, low self-esteem, and many other issues that the individual may not even realize are a result of their trauma. It can take a long time for a sense of safety to reappear in a person's life, but it can be done with patience.

Patience is a huge emphasis during this phase of recovery. In fact, Trauma Recovery (2013) uses the following metaphor to describe how this phase should be approached:

> The experience of emotional overwhelm is similar to that of a shaken bottle of soda. Inside the bottle is a tremendous amount of pressure. The safest way to release the pressure is to open and close the cap in a slow, cautious, and intentional manner so as to prevent an explosion.

When you are establishing your sense of safety and stabilization, be careful to take things slowly and don't push yourself. Begin with several days or weeks of self-care that makes you feel safe, such as using weighted blankets and watching reruns of your favorite shows. Make sure that you take care of yourself as you begin to release that pressure, or you will end up doing a lot of damage to your already shaky mindset.

Phase 2: Remembrance and Mourning

This is where a lot of the lessons we learned from Hall come into play. Many people will try to repress the grief and sadness that come along with abuse, but it is important to address those feelings before moving onto the next phase.

For many people, this phase is quite short. Even if it takes a long time for them to feel okay with releasing these feelings, once it is done, it is easy to recover from. For others, the grieving period can be rather long and can involve all five stages of the grieving process. Those stages are denial, anger, bargaining, depression, and finally, acceptance. You may notice yourself moving through all of those emotions as you come to terms with everything you have lost over the years, but you must give yourself the space to do so. Pushing these feelings aside will only cause them to explode sometime later, and it will inhibit your progress.

For this stage, writing about your feelings or watching emotional movies may be particularly helpful. Anything that allows you to express your feelings and come to terms with them is fantastic for processing grief.

Phase 3: Reconnection and Integration

This phase is where you might want to start including some of the harder self-care exercises we looked at earlier on in the chapter. You will feel the start of a new beginning, and you will have to approach this future head-on. This may mean creating new relationships, chasing new desires, and redefining who you are.

The trauma will still exist and may pop up from time to time. However, it will no longer be at the forefront of your mind, and it will not define everything you do. You will have the freedom to do that for yourself. Many people struggle with this phase of healing because they are unsure of who they are outside of their trauma, which is understandable and valid. Still, as long as you are patient and forgiving with yourself, you will forge yourself into someone that you respect and admire.

Many people in this stage benefit from peer mentoring or other services that allow them to continue growing and support them when they encounter any relapses. Some even want to go on with their professional therapy, even if their appointments are less frequent. This way, they can share new discoveries about themselves and learn to see the world through a lens unclouded by troublesome thoughts and anxieties. Even after your recovery is "complete," you may want to use counseling to help you tackle the everyday stressors of your adult life. Being in therapy is nothing to be ashamed of, and you don't need to be in a crisis to benefit from it.

Chapter 8:

Treating Narcissistic

Personality Disorder

For the final chapter of this book, we will discuss what clinical treatment of NPD looks like. I put this chapter last for a reason: "fixing" your sibling is not your responsibility. You should prioritize protecting yourself, healing yourself, and improving your own life. Still, if you would like to learn more about the techniques a therapist may use to help a narcissist recover from this condition, this chapter will be of great interest to you.

In fact, I think it may be helpful to have knowledge of these techniques so that you can use them in appropriate situations. While you should focus on keeping yourself safe, you can also try talking to your sibling with these clinical treatments in mind to make your interactions productive for both of you. Your sibling may get defensive or angry if you admit that these are skills you learned from studying therapy, but there are ways to incorporate these ideas subtly. I will give some pointers on how to incorporate these methods into casual interactions so that you don't endanger yourself when trying to help your sibling improve.

If you or your sibling is interested in pursuing therapy, you should contact therapists in your area and ask them about their experience with NPD. I will include a list of questions that you can ask a therapist to ensure that they will be a good fit for you, your sibling, and the rest of your family.

We will begin by talking about the general philosophy behind helping someone with NPD and then jump into specifics.

Therapy With Narcissistic Personality Disorder

As we have discussed already, most narcissists are extremely resistant to therapy. They either cannot believe that something is wrong with them, or they think of it as an insult. They may even be difficult to work with thanks to their manipulative and sometimes aggressive nature. The therapist must be ready to be manipulated and deal with aggressive behaviors, just as their other victims have. Moreover, the therapist must be ready to navigate the false self, an overall warped view of reality, and a number of potential comorbidities in order to truly help a narcissist. It is a long, difficult journey, but it can be worthwhile for both the patients and their loved ones.

Pietrangelo (2020) identifies seven steps that will likely be present in a narcissist's path to self-growth:

1. Overcoming the initial resistance to therapy
2. Recognizing narcissistic behaviors and how they negatively affect their daily life
3. Analyzing past experiences, traumas, or thoughts that may have given NPD the chance to develop
4. Understanding how these thought patterns affect others
5. Replacing distorted thoughts with a more realistic mindset
6. Exploring new patterns of thought and behavior and practicing them
7. Reflecting on the benefits of new behaviors

A number of things about these seven steps may stand out to you. For starters, it seems like it will take a very long time, and it often does. Some clients progress faster than others. However, when a person has lived with a narcissistic thought pattern for much of their lives, it will take some time to break it. Patience is important when treating a narcissist.

You may also notice that the concept of including other people is only introduced in step 4. It is easy to feel frustrated by this because you will want your sibling to realize as quickly as possible that they are hurting people, but this is a deliberate decision made by therapists across the world.

People with NPD do not feel empathy like a neurotypical person, so they struggle to comprehend any pain they may be causing others. It takes a little bit of build-up to get there, and introducing it too soon may cause a standstill. If you tell your narcissistic sibling, "Your behavior is a problem because it is hurting people," they are unlikely to understand or care and may want to cease therapy. To convince them that they have a problem, it is better to start off by looking at how their behaviors are self-sabotaging. Instead of saying, "You are hurting your brother," a therapist may say, "Your actions are causing you to conflict with your brother and miss out on a positive relationship with him." See how the sentiment is still focused on the narcissist? They will eventually come to understand how they inflict pain on others, but those steps are later in the process.

Steps 5 through 7 are focused on addressing and recovering from the false self. The narcissist has to go through the difficult journey of rediscovering themselves and sorting out what is a part of their false self versus their true self. Hence, they need to experiment with different personalities and see how they fit. Their therapist will encourage them to try new things, revisit old hobbies and activities from before the narcissistic traits set in (if such a thing is applicable), and try to rebuild themselves. This part of the healing process can take a long time.

It is important that the narcissist does not adopt the traits they are developing into a new false self. Thus, frequent check-ins are necessary to ensure that the effort is genuine. If it is forced and is accepted as part of the false self, they will have to find a new approach and start again.

Note that medication is not included in this seven-step journey. Medication is not a standard part of treatment for any of the 10 personality disorders in the DSM, but that does not necessarily mean that your sibling would receive no medication at all. Depending on their comorbidities, they may be prescribed medicine for depression, anxiety, OCD, or any other major mental disorder that hinders them from growing. For depression, they may receive a serotonin reuptake inhibitor (SSRI), such as fluoxetine, sertraline, or paroxetine. For those with uncontrollable mood swings, a mood stabilizer may be recommended, such as lithium. For symptoms related to anxiety, the patient may be prescribed any number of antipsychotic medicine (Cleveland Clinic, 2020). It is also possible that they would not be medicated at any point, and that is okay too. They can still change and improve from therapy alone, so don't fret!

According to Pietrangelo (2020), a professional will employ a number of techniques designed to help your sibling fulfill each step to self-growth with ease.

- **Psychotherapy:** This form of therapy is probably the type you picture when you think of a typical therapy session. It is also called talk therapy and involves exploring the reasons behind an emotion, thought, or behavior. It also often examines the past and how behaviors that were learned in childhood or adolescence can carry into adulthood and continue to affect us.

- **Cognitive behavioral therapy:** CBT is a type of therapy that is popular for clients with NPD. It typically includes homework assignments between sessions, which may range from journal entries, scheduling positive activities, creating artwork, and more. The aim is to identify unhealthy thoughts and replace them with something more productive, satisfying, and realistic. The homework assignments allow the patient to practice some of their new skills and report back to their therapist about how it went.

- **Schema therapy:** Schema therapy is a combination of psychotherapy and CBT and is extremely common in a clinical setting. Most likely, a patient will engage in both of these styles at the same time. For instance, they may complete their CBT activities on their own and then discuss their discoveries in psychotherapy the next time they see their therapist.

- **Gestalt therapy:** Although we traditionally think of therapy as being focused on examining the past, Gestalt therapy is centered on the present. The German word "gestalt" describes a pattern, so an individual's past is seen as the context of a current pattern. Through recognizing the present, a person will be encouraged to engage in more self-recognition and accountability.

- **Mentalization-based therapy:** MBT is focused on improving a person's ability to think about their own behaviors, as well as the possible thoughts and feelings of someone else. This method can be especially helpful for those with NPD because they may not have the innate ability to understand others, so this therapy will help introduce them to empathy. It will also encourage those who are more spontaneous and uncontrolled to sit back and think before they act.

- **Transference-focused psychotherapy:** In this form of therapy, the therapist takes on the role of an important figure in the patient's life and allows the patient to direct their feelings toward them. The therapist may be standing in for a parent, teacher, past lover, or anyone else whom the patient would benefit from talking to. Allowing them the space to yell, explain themselves, or simply talk will help create a sense of closure.

- **Dialectical behavior therapy:** DBT is a variance of CBT that is more centered on learning coping mechanisms. The homework assignments associated with this technique may include coping strategies, like practicing mindfulness, grounding, and other emotion regulation.

- **Metacognitive interpersonal therapy:** MIT encourages the eventual development of empathy and compassion by first looking at how interpersonal relationships can affect the self. It involves teaching the importance of communal unity, the ways in which our relationships can help us live fulfilling lives, and more. This type of therapy is key when working with a narcissist.

- **Eye movement desensitization and reprocessing (EMDR) therapy:** This is a type of therapy that redirects and distracts the brain while focusing on a traumatic event. By giving a person visual (and sometimes auditory) stimuli while encouraging them to envision and talk about trauma, the brain learns to associate the trauma with healing rather than pain. EMDR is an eight-step process that will hopefully lessen the strength of trauma and PTSD. This is especially helpful for narcissists who had a rough childhood.

Experiences With Therapy

Therapy looks different from person to person. Everyone will have a favorite style of treatment, as well as the least favorite, and it all depends on the individual's personality and preferences. Sometimes, it can be difficult to predict what will work best for a person, so it may take a bit of experimentation to figure out what will give the best results. It may also help to hear about real people's experiences with some of the different styles to get an idea of what they are like, who benefits from them, and what the downsides are.

The following four examples were posted online by people with NPD who have sought therapy or by loved ones of narcissists who have been in therapy. Although these examples do not touch on each of the treatment styles we discussed earlier, they give a bit of first-hand experience and some useful advice.

Example 1: Successful EMDR Treatment

Reddit user Turbophysics was raised by a psychopath, so he reports that his narcissism is rooted in trauma and rejection. Thankfully, he pursued therapy and had seen a lot of success, particularly when he used EMDR. Since EMDR is focused on redirecting trauma, it is no surprise that Turbophysics had a lot of success with this particular style of treatment. He started seeing positive effects after about six sessions of EMDR, each lasting around an hour.

He says, "I can't overstate how helpful therapy has been. I am not normal, but I am a new and better person that I actually like."

Example 2: 10 Years of Psychotherapy and CBT

Liquidstateofmind on Reddit has a friend who was diagnosed with NPD and has been in therapy for over 10 years. The friend has suffered a hard life full of childhood trauma. However, after a combination of psychotherapy and CBT, he started regaining control of his life. It has been three years of consistent sessions, and he has been improving ever since. He finds the psychotherapy a bit more helpful than the CBT, but the two styles seem to work well in tandem to help him make a complete and full recovery.

Example 3: Insight on Schema Therapies

User Ntheway on Reddit reports using a number of schema exercises during her time in therapy, and they have been very helpful. She has a word of advice for those who may be seeking schema therapy: "The trick is to not drop out ... no matter how uncomfortable it gets." Therapy can be uncomfortable for everyone, but it is especially challenging for narcissists because it aims to change the way they have seen themselves and the world around them for years. Ntheway also thinks that the dropout rate of schema therapy is very high, even though the sessions can be extremely beneficial if the person sticks with it. If schema therapy is too overwhelming, she recommends pursuing a technique that is not talk-focused, such as EMDR or touch therapy.

Example 4: Lifelong Treatment and New Revelations

Redditor Plus_Wallaby2937 is an older sufferer of NPD who has been retired for a few years. He is 66 years old and reports that therapy is often a lifelong process, but it can be very worthwhile so long as there is trust between the patient and therapist. Because he decided to stick with therapy through all of these years, he has seen a lot of improvement and no longer feels like "two people" inside—the false self and the true self. He has also recognized the cause of his narcissism, which was not clear at first, and is making sense of his life. He now states he has a 99 percent understanding of everything that happened in his life, which is an impressive feat considering the dissociation and confabulation involved in NPD. He does not share a favorite style of therapy but seems confident that if a therapist is genuine, caring, and easy to talk to, the sessions will be helpful in the long run.

Pursuing Therapy

Finding a therapist who is qualified to handle both NPD or C-PTSD and also compatible with your (or your sibling's) personality is a frustrating and often nerve-wracking endeavor. You might not expect it to be very difficult, but it can actually feel very hopeless sometimes. Even Jeff Guenther, a licensed professional counselor in Portland, Oregon, admits that it can be unusually hard to start therapy. "As a therapist myself," he says, "I want to apologize on behalf of the mental health community. I am truly sorry about how annoying and bizarrely difficult it is to find a mental health counselor" (Guenther, 2018). However, he promises that he has advice that will help make the process a little bit easier.

Finding a Good Therapist

As Guenther explains, one main reason why finding a therapist is so difficult is that people don't typically talk about how great their counselor is. Unfortunately, our society frowns upon seeking help for mental health issues, so the issue is fairly hush-hush. It also does not help that therapy is such a personal matter that one person's favorite therapist might be their cousin's least favorite, so referrals are unlikely to be very helpful anyway.

So you will be left doing the searching and calling for yourself. One of the most confusing things you will encounter is that of credentials and licenses. Although that side of the story may seem overwhelming, Guenther says that it should not be a major source of stress. It should not even be a deciding factor when you pick your therapist! Guenther (2018) explains it best:

> As far as you (the average therapy seeker) should be concerned, a licensed professional counselor (LPC) is the same as a licensed marriage and family therapist (LMFT), which is the same as a licensed clinical social worker (LCSW). All those therapists are masters-level therapists, which means they have a master's degree in the counseling field and they are licensed in their state to treat clients.

To be qualified to counsel and take on clients of their own, therapists have to undergo a large amount of field experience under a supervisor, take an exam at the end of their fieldwork to prove their knowledge, and register themselves with their state board. All in all, it takes between two and five years to be certified. That means therapists with those fancy titles are very much qualified to talk to you, your sibling, or both of you. If you are comfortable, you can consider seeking out someone who is currently getting their field experience. They typically offer lower prices, and they also talk to their supervisor about your case (while maintaining confidentiality, of course), so you will have a team of therapists helping you out.

The easiest way to find a therapist is through a Google search, which Guenther says is a perfectly fine method, but he has a few tips. First of all, he wants you to be very specific in the search bar. Do not simply search "therapists in New York." Search "therapists specializing in trauma recovery in New York." He also advises that you look beyond the first page in your search. The first results are not necessarily the best therapists—they are just the best at understanding search engines and using key terms. Don't be afraid to click on the second and third pages of your search results.

If you would rather hear recommendations from people you know, there are a few ways to do so. Your doctor and insurance provider can provide some recommendations, so that can give you a decent starting point. You can also try asking your friends and family if they know anyone; you might be surprised at who has been going to therapy!

Questions to Ask a Potential Therapist

Think of your quest for a therapist as one of those cheesy dating games. Before you dive head-first into a long-term relationship, you will want to ask a few questions about how they prefer to communicate and what their "type" is and maybe learn if they trigger any of your pet peeves, right? The same goes for a therapist. It is completely acceptable to ask a potential therapist a bunch of questions over the phone before you decide if they are a good fit for you. It is better to ask than risk setting yourself (or your sibling) with someone who will not accomplish what you are looking for. Hence, it is a good idea to have a few questions in mind as you begin searching for therapists.

I have a few suggestions about questions to ask. It may be a good idea to keep this page in front of you as you call, or you can have them written down on a separate paper.

1. Have you worked with NPD clients before?

This question is key. Clients with NPD offer a lot of unique issues and can sometimes place a lot of stress on a therapist, so you must know whether they have the know-how to deal with that. You may also want to ask if they have experience with any of your sibling's comorbidities, such as alcoholism, substance abuse, or anything else that you feel would come up in therapy.

2. Have you worked with a variety of NPD types and subtypes?

Communicating with a classic narcissist looks extremely different from communicating with a vulnerable narcissist, so just being familiar with one of the types is not going to cut it. This question will help you gauge the scope of the therapist's experience and ensure that they know what they are doing. Because of confidentiality, they may not be able to give you a detailed explanation of all the types they have worked with, but they can give you a simple yes or no that will help you decide if they have the experience you are looking for.

3. When was the last time you worked with someone who has NPD?

Many people won't mind that their therapist has not talked to someone with NPD in over 15 years, but for others, it is a deal-breaker. If they say that they have not had an NPD client in a long time, a good follow-up question would be "Have you been keeping up to date with the recent literature?" With the ways technology and social media have been affected by the disorder, it is incredibly important for a therapist to stay up-to-date.

4. Who is your ideal client, especially in terms of NPD?

To answer this question, your therapist may tell you which type or subtype they are the most experienced with. This will help you decide which therapist is the best fit. Although your sibling may not be the therapist's exact ideal client, the closer you can get, the better!

5. How long have you been practicing?

Some people prefer a therapist who has been in the field for a long time, while others prefer to talk to someone a bit younger. It all comes down to personal preference. Either way, this question will help you gain some more information about the therapist that may assist you when making the final decision.

6. What is your general approach to helping?

This is an open-ended question that can be answered in a number of different ways. The therapist may begin talking about their communication style, how demanding or lenient they are, or their broad philosophy toward the position. Regardless of how they decide to answer, it will tell you a lot about the treatment styles they prefer. You may hear something you really like, or you may hear something that you know won't work.

7. What is a successful session to you?

Here, the therapist may tell you about what a typical session looks like or the sort of techniques they use and prefer. They may also simply tell you that a successful session is one where the client makes progress. Knowing their specific goals for each individual session will tell you what to expect when the sessions begin, letting you focus less on the therapist's expectations and more on personal growth.

8. Are you certified in ___?

This question is especially helpful if there is a certain technique or style that you want to try. Some treatments, such as EMDR, require a special certification, so it is worthwhile to ask if someone is qualified to perform it if that is important to you.

Don't limit yourself to those eight questions! Before you call, take a moment to consider what is important to you in a therapist. Consider the therapist's gender, race, views on sexuality and sex, or other things that are important to you or your sibling. You may think of plenty more questions for your potential therapist. Don't be afraid to ask. They want to ensure that you are as comfortable as possible, so these questions will likely be helpful for both of you.

Knowing if a Therapist Is Good for You

This is the hard part. After you have searched for therapists and called a few of them, you will have to make a decision. Guenther has a few more suggestions for this stage of your decision as well. First of all, you should weigh the options based on their specialties. You must know whether or not they offer the techniques you are hoping for. However, there is more to a therapist than just that. You should also enjoy their personality and feel safe talking to them. Guenther says that most therapists put a lot of information on their personal web pages and blogs, so reading through those can be a good way for you to get to know the kind of person they are. Look at those pages and consider your preferences. Would you rather talk to someone who is nurturing or someone who will be more like a doctor with you? Is there a gender you feel safer opening up to? Do you want them to be older than you or a little closer to your age? Do you prefer someone who is funny and will joke with you or someone who will help you take your problems seriously?

Finally, it can be a good idea to request a free consultation. Most therapists will allow you to talk to them for free for a few minutes, whether you can do so in person or over the phone. Either way, having a real conversation with them will definitely help you judge whether or not they have the energy you need (Guenther, 2020).

Tips for Therapy

When seeking therapy, there will probably be a few nerves involved before that first session. Even though the concept of seeking counseling has been destigmatized over the years, it is still a little scary to think about sitting down with a stranger and spilling your heart to them. It is natural to fear judgment, miscommunication, and other complications that might make your appointment a bit difficult to deal with, especially when you are potentially dealing with trust issues associated with your trauma. No one expects a therapist (or a client!) to be perfect, but there are a few things you can do to make sure that the sessions go as smoothly as possible.

Here are a few tips for you to keep in mind as you begin therapy, or you can give these pieces of advice to your sibling if they are about to start.

1. If you don't like something your therapist is doing, let them know. They want to help you in the most efficient way possible, so if they are doing something that is not working, they will want you to tell them. Being honest is a good way to make sure no one's time is being wasted. You may feel a little rude when you give your therapist criticism, but it is actually advantageous to everyone.

2. Think of therapy as a 24/7 journey. It is good to put in some effort during your sessions, but most of the work will be done outside of the office. Take the lessons you learn in therapy and work on applying them in your daily life, even outside of your assigned work. Your therapist will be excited to hear about your progress!

3. Value the process. It is easy to get impatient for results. Although it is good to look forward to doing better, it will be hard to stick with it if you are only looking for changes in behavior. Start valuing the act of improving yourself, even if the improvements have not come yet.

4. Schedule your appointments for a good time. You may think you can go to work 30 minutes after your session, but it will actually be a good idea to give yourself some time afterward so that you can process, accept, and think. Some sessions might dig up triggering and upsetting

memories, so give yourself some space when that happens.

5. Be as odd as you need to be. Did your therapist say something that brought up a memory from fourth grade? Let them know! Sudden impulses, thoughts, daydreams, fantasies, and urges can sometimes tell us a lot about ourselves. Your therapist will be extremely interested to hear them when they come up. Speak freely and mention anything that might be on your mind.

6. Ask away! Some people think that they are not the ones asking questions during a session, but it is actually a two-way street. If you don't understand something your therapist is saying, ask them to clarify. They want to ensure that you are fully on-board with what they are saying. Hence, you are actually doing them a favor by letting them know where you are so that they can meet you there.

7. Keep your eyes off the clock. When you are stressing about how much time is left in a session, you may not be fully engaged in the conversation. Your therapist will be responsible for wrapping up on time, so you don't have to give it a second thought. They will let you know when time is up!

8. You don't have to tell your friends about your sessions if you don't want to. Your therapy is

for you and you alone, so it's okay if you don't want to send the details to your group chat if that is not your style. You don't owe information to your family, either, so don't let them pressure you into giving specifics over dinner. Therapy can be a completely private endeavor for many, and you have a right to keep your discoveries to yourself.

9. Think of your first appointment as an interview, not a session. If you enter the therapist's office for the first time and expect to immediately start talking about the core of your problems, you are going to be sorely disappointed. The first session is typically spent on introductions, goal setting, and possibly establishing the context of why you have decided to start therapy. You are extremely unlikely to start discussing your feelings on the first day, so there is no need to stress about that right off the bat.

10. If you decide that you want to switch therapists, end therapy in general, or leave in any capacity, let your therapist know. They will not be offended. It happens all the time, and they know you are simply making the best decision for yourself at the time. If you give them a heads-up that you plan on leaving, they will probably want to celebrate everything you have

done so far and invite you to reflect on the journey, which can be an enlightening activity that you won't want to miss out on.

Conclusion

You have gone through a lot. You have been belittled and controlled in your childhood when you were supposed to be growing and learning. Instead of learning how to navigate the world and be successful, you learned to live in fear. You developed several trauma responses and habits that kept you safe from abuse and taught you to be okay with loneliness and be at peace with being the "lesser sibling." You might have fallen victim to triangularization, which made you feel less important than other people. Perhaps you have been gaslighted into thinking that you committed some great offense against your sibling when you were actually just offering criticism or standing up for yourself. Living with a narcissist may leave you with many emotional wounds that you may not have even been aware of, and it may take you some time to fully recover from everything that has been done to you.

However, you are not powerless. You have decided to educate yourself and learn about NPD, and you have certainly learned a lot! You have learned about the history of the disorder and what it means to obtain the diagnosis. You have learned how NPD can develop and how environmental versus inherited behaviors can affect an individual. You have learned about the three types and two subtypes of narcissism, how they are defined, and how to identify what kind of narcissist your sibling is. You can now identify the cycle of narcissistic abuse and recognize where you stand in the cycle, as well as what forms of abuse your sibling tends to use. You also understand the ins and outs of the disorder, such as the false self, dissociation, comorbidities, and the narcissist's brain structure. Besides that, you have encountered so many real-life examples of people dealing with narcissists that you now understand how common your situation is. You are not alone, and many people can help you.

Moreover, if you choose to, you can use the techniques suggested in this book to break free of the cycle and improve your life. You know how to set boundaries, go no contact, and interact with your sibling with a new mindset. You know how to use self-care, grounding techniques, self-talk, and other healing activities to help yourself move on from this painful chapter of your life. Most significantly, you know how to track your progress.

You have learned what it means to receive professional therapy and are familiar with several styles of treatment. Moreover, you know how a therapist would treat your sibling if they also seek professional help. You have everything you need. You already took the first step by doing the research. Now you just need to stick with it and turn your knowledge into action.

As I have stated in the beginning of this book, my ultimate aim is to pass on the information I have learned about NPD from my own attempts to free myself from a narcissist's grasp. Everything I have taught you was obtained from five long years of intensive study, experiments, and first-hand experience. It was a hard road, and it would be selfish of me not to pass on my discoveries to someone else who might benefit from it.

As I finish out the final paragraphs of this book, I find myself feeling very satisfied. I have already said everything I possibly could to be helpful, and I have the utmost faith that everyone who has read this book from start to finish is prepared to start a new life. You may still be feeling nervous, and that is understandable. You are in a scary situation, and the prospect of starting a new chapter can be very intimidating. However, even if you are not confident in yourself, I am confident in your abilities, and I know you can do great things.

Allow me to leave you with a few truths that you can feel free to use as affirmations or self-talk if they resonate with you: You are not to blame. You have endured a lot, and you are very strong. You are extremely knowledgeable and prepared to defend yourself. You are not alone. You are worthy. You are good.

If you enjoyed this book, please consider leaving a review on Amazon and giving it a positive rating so that it can find more people who will benefit from its contents. I wish you luck in all of your future endeavors, and I hope that these difficulties are soon a thing of the past.

References

Abela, J., & Hankin, B. (2008). *Cognitive vulnerability to depression in children and adolescents: A developmental psychopathology perspective.* American Psychological Association. https://psycnet.apa.org/record/2008-01178-003

Adamo, N. (2020). *The no contact rule: How to make it easier & more effective.* https://natashaadamo.com/no-contact-rule/

American Journal of Psychiatry (2006). *Genetic and environmental contributions to dimensions of personality disorder.* https://ajp.psychiatryonline.org/doi/abs/10.1176/ajp.150.12.1826

Badminton, N. (2020). *The future of life in America: 2020 report.* Intensions Consulting. https://www.intensions.co/future-of-life-america-2020

Bailey, R. (2020). *What does the cerebral cortex do?* ThoughtCo. https://www.thoughtco.com/anatomy-of-the-brain-cerebral-cortex-373217

Bartosch, J. (2020). *Study shows narcissistic personality disorder may have a biological component.* UChicago Medicine.
https://www.uchicagomedicine.org/forefront/research-and-discoveries-articles/study-shows-narcissistic-personality-disorder-may-have-a-biological-component

Beauty After Bruises (2018). *4 tools to cope with flashbacks.*
https://www.beautyafterbruises.org/blog/flashbacks

Beauty After Bruises (2019). *Self-care 101: Featuring 101 self-care techniques for trauma survivors.*
https://www.beautyafterbruises.org/blog/selfcare

Behavioral Health Florida (2020). *The three clusters of personality disorders.* Behavioral Health.
https://www.behavioralhealthflorida.com/blog/three-clusters-personality-disorders/

Bloudoff-Indelicato, M. (2016). *The 14 questions you should ask a therapist before your first appointment.* Washingtonian.
https://www.washingtonian.com/2016/03/03/the-14-questions-you-must-ask-a-therapist-before-your-first-appointment/

Bridges to Recovery (n.d.). *Narcissistic personality disorder treatment.*
https://www.bridgestorecovery.com/narcissisti

c-personality-disorder/narcissistic-personality-disorder-treatment/

Burgemeester, A. (2020, April 24). *Is Narcissism Genetic? The Narcissistic Life.* https://thenarcissisticlife.com/is-narcissism-genetic/

Caligor, E., Levy, K. N., & Yeomans, F. E. (2015). *Narcissistic personality disorder: Diagnostic and clinical challenges.* American Journal of Psychiatry. https://ajp.psychiatryonline.org/doi/full/10.11 76/appi.ajp.2014.14060723

Campell, K., & Crist, C. (2020, October 6). *How narcissism and leadership go hand-in-hand.* Psychology Today. https://www.psychologytoday.com/us/blog/n ew-science-narcissism/202010/how-narcissism-and-leadership-go-hand-in-hand

Cartwright, M. (2017). *Narcissus.* Ancient. https://www.ancient.eu/Narcissus/

Charité-Universitätsmedizin Berlin (2013). *Altered brain structure in pathological narcissism.* Science Daily. https://www.sciencedaily.com/releases/2013/0 6/130619101434.htm

Charité-Universitätsmedizin Berlin (2013). *Altered brain structure in pathological narcissism.* Science Daily. www.sciencedaily.com/releases/2013/06/1306 19101434.htm

Cleveland Clinic (2020). *Narcissistic personality disorder management and treatment.* https://my.clevelandclinic.org/health/diseases/9742-narcissistic-personality-disorder/management-and-treatment

Davies, J. (2017). *9 famous narcissists in history and today's world.* Learning Mind. https://www.learning-mind.com/famous-narcissists/

Eddy, B. (2018). *3 ways to spot a narcissist.* Psychology Today. https://www.psychologytoday.com/us/blog/5-types-people-who-can-ruin-your-life/201808/3-ways-spot-narcissist

Edershile, E. A., & Wright, A. G. C. (2020). *Fluctuations in grandiose and vulnerable narcissist states: A momentary perspective.* UChicago Medicine. https://www.uchicagomedicine.org/forefront/research-and-discoveries-articles/study-shows-narcissistic-personality-disorder-may-have-a-biological-component

Elgan, M. (2009). *Does mobile and social technology breed narcissism?* InfoWorld. https://www.infoworld.com/article/2630877/does-mobile-and-social-technology-breed-narcissism-.html

George, F. R. (2018). *The cognitive neuroscience of narcissism.* Journal of Brain, Behaviour and Cognitive Sciences.

https://www.imedpub.com/articles/the-cognitive-neuroscience-of-narcissism.php?aid=22149

Greenberg, E. (2020). *Have you been the victim of narcissistic triangulation?* Psychology Today. https://www.psychologytoday.com/us/blog/understanding-narcissism/202008/have-you-been-the-victim-narcissistic-triangulation

Guenther, J. (2018). *A beginners guide to therapy (part 1): How to find a therapist.* TherapyDen. https://www.therapyden.com/blog/a-beginners-guide-to-therapy-how-to-find-a-therapist

Hall, J. L. (2019). *6 core insights from a narcissistic abuse recovery coach.* Psychology Today. https://www.psychologytoday.com/us/blog/the-narcissist-in-your-life/201911/6-core-insights-narcissistic-abuse-recovery-coach

Johnson, E. B. (2020). *Safeguarding yourself from narcissistic rage.* Medium. https://medium.com/lady-vivra/safeguarding-yourself-from-narcissistic-rage-f93c64de2869

Kendell, R. (2018). *The distinction between personality disorder and mental illness.* The British Journal of Psychiatry. https://www.cambridge.org/core/journals/the-british-journal-of-psychiatry/article/distinction-between-

personality-disorder-and-mental-
illness/F4FC446AEB38B5704ED132245F86E9
3B

Kennedy, M. (2020). *The difference between CPTSD and PTSD and how to treat each condition.* Insider. https://www.insider.com/cptsd-vs-ptsd

Kluger, J. (2019). *The best and worst narcissists in world history.* Big Think. https://bigthink.com/videos/does-the-white-house-attract-narcissists-with-jeffrey-kluger

Lampitt, C. (2019). *Detecting and healing from narcissistic abuse.* Resolve. https://www.kcresolve.com/blog/detecting-and-healing-from-narcissistic-abuse.

Lancer, D. (2017). *How to spot narcissistic abuse.* Psychology Today. https://www.psychologytoday.com/us/blog/toxic-relationships/201709/how-spot-narcissistic-abuse

Lazarus, R. (1993, February). *From Psychological Stress to the Emotions: A History of Changing Outlooks.* Annual Reviews. https://www.annualreviews.org/doi/10.1146/annurev.ps.44.020193.000245

Lessons from History (2020). *When narcissists rule.* Medium. https://medium.com/lessons-from-history/when-narcissists-rule-a15b998f6960

Li, P. (2020). *Diathesis stress model: Psychology.* Parenting For Brain. https://www.parentingforbrain.com/diathesis-stress-model/

Loudis, J. (2018). *Editor's note: Megalomania.* World Policy Journal. https://read.dukeupress.edu/world-policy-journal/article/35/2/1/134856/Editor-s-NoteMegalomania.

Luo, Y. L. L., Cai, H., & Song, H. (2014). *A behavioral genetic study of intrapersonal and interpersonal dimensions of narcissism.* PloS one. https://www.ncbi.nlm.nih.gov/pmc/articles/PMC3973692/

Mayo Clinic (2018). *Persistent depressive disorder (dysthymia).* https://www.mayoclinic.org/diseases-conditions/persistent-depressive-disorder/symptoms-causes/syc-20350929

Mind (2017). *What is complex PTSD?* https://www.mind.org.uk/information-support/types-of-mental-health-problems/post-traumatic-stress-disorder-ptsd/complex-ptsd/

Narcissist Abuse Support. (2019). *What type of supply were you that attracted a narcissist?* https://narcissistabusesupport.com/what-type-of-narcissistic-supply-were-you/

National Institute of Mental Health (2017). *Borderline personality disorder.*

https://www.nimh.nih.gov/health/topics/bord
erline-personality-disorder/index.shtml

Nenadic, I., Güllmar, D., Dietzek, M., Langbein, K., Steinke, J., & Gaser, C. (2015). Brain structure in narcissistic personality disorder: a VBM and DTI pilot study. *Psychiatry research*, *231*(2), 184–186.
https://doi.org/10.1016/j.pscychresns.2014.11.001

NPR (2007). *Study sees rise in narcissism among students.* https://www.npr.org/templates/story/story.php?storyId=7618722%3FstoryId

O'Reilly, C. A., & Hall, N. (2021). *Grandiose narcissists and decision making: Impulsive, overconfident, and skeptical of experts-but seldom in doubt.* Science Direct.
https://www.sciencedirect.com/science/article/abs/pii/S0191886920304694?via%3Dihub

Paris, J. (2014). *Modernity and Narcissistic Personality Disorder.* American Psychological Association. https://psycnet.apa.org/doiLanding?doi=10.1037%2Fa0028580

Pietrangelo, A. (2020). *What therapy for narcissism involves: Steps and what to expect.* Healthline. https://www.healthline.com/health/therapy-for-narcissism

Psychology Today (2019). *Narcissistic Personality Disorder.*
https://www.psychologytoday.com/us/conditi
ons/narcissistic-personality-disorder

Radin, S. (2019). *How to create boundaries with a toxic family
member.* Allure.
https://www.allure.com/story/toxic-family-
how-create-boundaries

Ranch TN (2013). *Brain abnormalities found in narcissists.*
Recovery Ranch.
https://www.recoveryranch.com/addiction-
blog/brain-abnormalities-found-in-narcissists/

Robitz, R. (2018). *What are personality disorders?* American
Psychiatric Association.
https://www.psychiatry.org/patients-
families/personality-disorders/what-are-
personality-disorders

Rosglas Recovery (2019). *Signs and symptoms of narcissistic
abuse syndrome.*
https://www.rosglasrecovery.com/signs-and-
symptoms-of-narcissistic-abuse-syndrome/.

Schulze, L., Dziobek, I., Vater, A., Heekeren, H. R.,
Bajbouj, M., Renneberg, B., Heuser, I., &
Roepke, S. (2013). Gray matter abnormalities in
patients with narcissistic personality disorder.
Journal of Psychiatric Research, 47(10), 1363–1369.
https://doi.org/10.1016/j.jpsychires.2013.05.01
7

Stinson, F., Dawson, D., Goldstein, R., Chou, S., Huang, B., Smith, S., & Grant, B. (2008). *Prevalence, correlates, disability, and comorbidity of DSM-IV narcissistic personality disorder: Results from the wave 2 national epidemiologic survey on alcohol and related conditions.* NCBI. https://www.ncbi.nlm.nih.gov/pmc/articles/PMC2669224/

Torgersen, S., Myers, J., Reichborn-Kjennerud, T., Røysamb, E., Kubarych, T. S., & Kendler, K. S. (2012). *The heritability of Cluster B personality disorders assessed both by personal interview and questionnaire.* Journal of personality disorders, 26(6), 848–866. https://doi.org/10.1521/pedi.2012.26.6.848

Trauma Recovery (2013). *Phases of trauma recovery.* https://trauma-recovery.ca/recovery/phases-of-trauma-recovery/

Vaknin, S. (2018). *Dr. Jackal and Mr. Hide (somatic vs. cerebral narcissists).* Healthy Place. https://www.healthyplace.com/personality-disorders/malignant-self-love/dr-jackal-and-mr-hide-somatic-vs-cerebral-narcissists

Vaknin, S. (2020). *Dissociation and confabulation in narcissistic disorders.* Herald Open Access. https://www.heraldopenaccess.us/openaccess/dissociation-and-confabulation-in-narcissistic-disorders

Printed in the USA
CPSIA information can be obtained
at www.ICGtesting.com
LVHW010504311223
767720LV00084B/2973

9 781087 943862